The best learned words in medicine!

D0846660

Medical Terminology
Flashcards

Second Edition

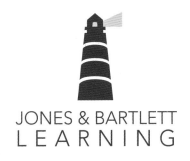

JONES & BARTLETT
LEARNING

World Headquarters
Jones & Bartlett Learning
5 Wall Street
Burlington, MA 01803
978-443-5000
info@jblearning.com
www.jblearning.com

Jones & Bartlett Learning books and products are available through most bookstores and online booksellers. To contact Jones & Bartlett Learning directly, call 800-832-0034, fax 978-443-8000, or visit our website, www.jblearning.com.

Substantial discounts on bulk quantities of Jones & Bartlett Learning publications are available to corporations, professional associations, and other qualified organizations. For details and specific discount information, contact the special sales department at Jones & Bartlett Learning via the above contact information or send an email to specialsales@jblearning.com.

26810-2

Production Credits

VP, Product Management: Amanda Martin
Director of Product Management: Cathy L. Esperti
Product Specialist: Ashley Malone
Product Coordinator: Elena Sorrentino
Project Manager: Lori Mortimer
Digital Project Specialist: Angela Dooley
Director of Marketing: Andrea DeFronzo
Marketing Manager: Suzy Balk
Production Services Manager: Colleen Lamy

VP, Manufacturing and Inventory Control: Therese Connell
Product Fulfillment Manager: Wendy Kilborn
Composition: S4Carlisle Publishing Services
Project Management: S4Carlisle Publishing Services
Cover & Text Design: Briana Yates
Senior Media Development Editor: Troy Liston
Rights Specialist: Rebecca Damon
Printing and Binding: LSC Communications

Library of Congress Cataloging-in-Publication Data
Library of Congress Cataloging-in-Publication Data unavailable at time of printing.

6048

Printed in the United States of America
24 23 22 21 20   10 9 8 7 6 5 4 3 2 1

Brief Overview

Medical Terminology Flashcards, **Second Edition** contains 800 flashcards made up of prefixes, suffixes, and root words to help users learn the building blocks of medical terminology. Each form is presented on the front of the card, and the definition and word building samples appear on the back. This edition features a new full-color design with specialties color-coded and illustrations added to cards. Any student of medical terminology, or any student in nursing, health professions, or medicine will value this quick, easy format for assessing their medical terminology knowledge.

How to Use

Medical Terminology Flashcards, Second Edition has been updated to a new, easy-to-use format. Students can choose to use this bound and perforated study tool in various ways, either as a book or by tearing the pages out and creating their own flashcards.

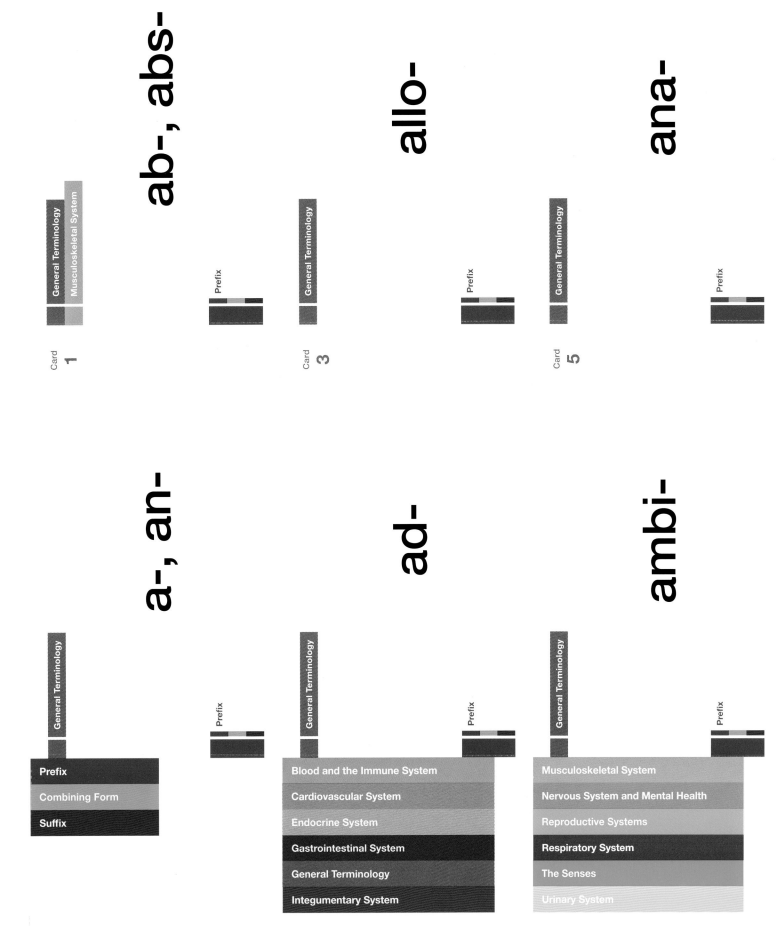

from, away from, off

aborad
(ab-or-ad)

In a direction away from the mouth

Word Building Example:

---

other, differing from normal

allograft
(allo-graft)

A graft transplanted between genetically nonidentical individuals of the same species.

Word Building Example:

cables

segmental
allograft

curved
washer

---

up, toward, apart

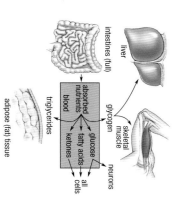

liver

intestines (full)

adipose (fat) tissue

triglycerides

absorbed
nutrients
blood

glycogen

skeletal
muscle

glucose
fatty acids
ketones

neurons

all
cells

---

anabolism
(ana-bol-ism)

The building up in the body of complex chemical compounds from smaller simpler compounds (e.g., proteins from amino acids), usually with the use of energy.

Word Building Example:

---

not, without, less

anaerophyte
(an-aero-phyte)

A plant that grows without air.

Word Building Example:

---

increase, adherence, to, toward

adduction
(ad-duct-ion)

Movement of a body part toward the median plane (of the body, in the case of limbs; of the hand or foot, in the case of digits) or midline of the body.

Word Building Example:

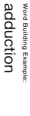

adduction

abduction

adduction

abduction

medial
rotation

lateral
rotation

lateral
rotation

medial
rotation

---

around, both, both sides

ambidextrous
(ambi-dextr-ous)

Having equal facility in the use of both hands.

Word Building Example:

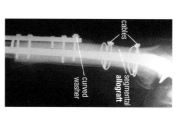

anti-

General Terminology

ante-

General Terminology

Prefix

Prefix

Combining Form

Suffix

auto-

General Terminology

Prefix

apo-

General Terminology

Prefix

Blood and the Immune System

Cardiovascular System

Endocrine System

Gastrointestinal System

General Terminology

Integumentary System

bio-

General Terminology

Prefix

bi-

General Terminology

Prefix

Musculoskeletal System

Nervous System and Mental Health

Reproductive Systems

Respiratory System

The Senses

Urinary System

against, opposing

antibiotic
(anti-bio-tic)

Denotes any substance that acts against susceptible microorganisms.

Word Building Example:

---

self, same

autosome
(auto-some)

Any chromosome other than a sex chromosome; autosomes normally occur in pairs in somatic cells and singly in gametes.

Word Building Example:

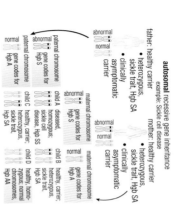

autosomal recessive gene inheritance
example: Sickle cell disease

father: healthy carrier
- heterozygous, sickle trait, Hgb SA
- clinically asymptomatic carrier

mother: healthy carrier
- heterozygous, sickle trait, Hgb SA
- clinically asymptomatic carrier

paternal chromosome gene codes for Hgb S — abnormal
paternal chromosome gene codes for Hgb A — normal

maternal chromosome gene codes for Hgb S — abnormal
maternal chromosome gene codes for Hgb A — normal

child A: diseased, homozygous, sickle cell disease, Hgb SS — abnormal abnormal

child B: healthy, carrier, heterozygous, sickle trait, Hgb SA — abnormal normal

child C: healthy carrier, heterozygous, sickle trait, Hgb SA — normal abnormal

child D: healthy, homozygous; normal chromosomes, Hgb AA — normal normal

---

life

---

against, opposing

---

before, in front of, forward

antenatal
(ante-nat-al)

Preceding birth.

Word Building Example:

---

separated from, derived from

apobiosis
(apo-bi-osis)

Death, especially local death of a part of the organism.

Word Building Example:

---

twice, double

biceps
(bi-ceps)

A muscle with two origins or heads. Commonly used to refer to the biceps brachii muscle.

Word Building Example:

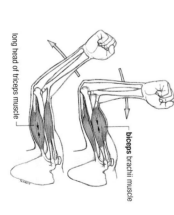

long head of triceps muscle

biceps brachii muscle

---

biology
(bio-logy)

The science concerned with the phenomena of life and

Word Building Example:

brady-

Cardiovascular System

brachy-

General Terminology

Prefix

Combining Form

Suffix

Prefix

cata-

General Terminology

Prefix

caci-, caco-

General Terminology

Prefix

Blood and the Immune System

Cardiovascular System

Endocrine System

Gastrointestinal System

General Terminology

Integumentary System

cero-, cerumin/o

The Senses

Prefix

centi-

General Terminology

Prefix

Musculoskeletal System

Nervous System and Mental Health

Reproductive Systems

Respiratory System

The Senses

Urinary System

slow

bradycardia
(brady-card-ia)

Slowness of the heartbeat, usually a rate less than 60 beats per minute.

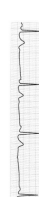

short

brachycephaly
(brachy-cephal-ic)

Shortness or broadness of the head.

Word Building Example:

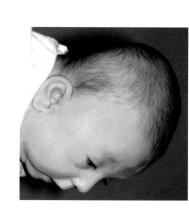

---

down

intestines (empty)

liver
glycogen

blood
glucose
triglycerides
adipose (fat tissue)
fatty acids
ketones
neurons
all cells

catabolism
(cata-bol-ism)

The breaking down in the body of complex chemical compounds into simpler ones (e.g., glycogen to CO_2 and H_2O), often accompanied by the liberation of energy.

Word Building Example:

bad, ill

cacogeusia
(caco-geusia)

A bad taste due to a bad-tasting substance, uncinate epilepsy, or a delusion.

Word Building Example:

---

wax

ceruminolytic
(cerumino-lytic)

One of several substances instilled into the external auditory canal to soften wax.

Word Building Example:

one hundredth

centile
(centi-ile)

One hundredth.

Word Building Example:

cin-, cine-

General Terminology

Prefix

chord-

General Terminology

Prefix

Prefix
Combining Form
Suffix

con-, com-

General Terminology

Prefix

circum-

General Terminology

Prefix

Blood and the Immune System
Cardiovascular System
Endocrine System
Gastrointestinal System
General Terminology
Integumentary System

copro-

Gastrointestinal System

Prefix

contra-

General Terminology

Prefix

Musculoskeletal System
Nervous System and Mental Health
Reproductive Systems
Respiratory System
The Senses
Urinary System

movement

Word Building Example:

cineradiography
(cine-radio-graphy)

Radiography of an organ in motion, e.g., the heart, the gastrointestinal tract.

cord

Word Building Example:

chorditis
(chord-itis)

Inflammation of a cord; usually a vocal cord.

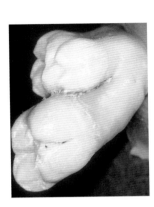

with, together,
in association

circular, circular movement

Word Building Example:

concrescence
(con-crescence)

1. Fusion of originally separate parts. 2. The union of the roots of two adjacent teeth by cementum.

Word Building Example:

circumduction
(circum-duct-ion)

Movement of a body part, e.g., a limb, in a circular direction.

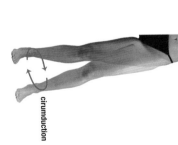

circumduction

feces

opposed, against

Word Building Example:

coproantibodies
(copro-anti-bodies)

Antibodies found in the intestine and in feces...

Word Building Example:

contraindication
(contra-indication)

Any special symptom or circumstance that renders the use of a remedy or the carrying out of a procedure inadvisable, due to risk.

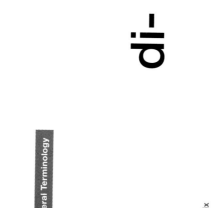
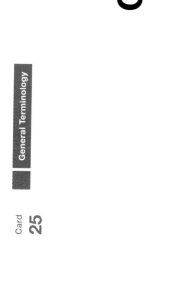
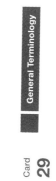
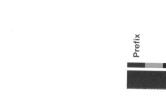
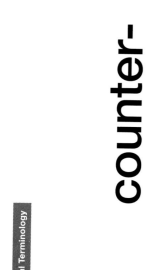
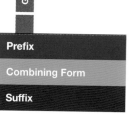
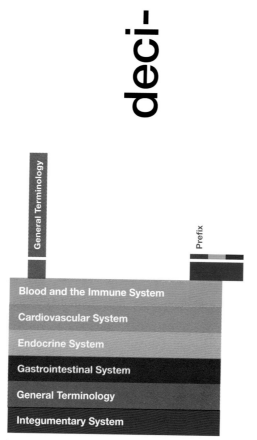
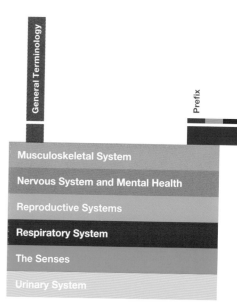

Card 26

de-

General Terminology

Card 25

counter-

General Terminology

Prefix

Combining Form

Suffix

Card 28

di-

Prefix

General Terminology

Card 27

deci-

Prefix

General Terminology

Blood and the Immune System

Cardiovascular System

Endocrine System

Gastrointestinal System

General Terminology

Integumentary System

Card 30

dis-

Prefix

Card 29

dia-

Prefix

General Terminology

Musculoskeletal System

Nervous System and Mental Health

Reproductive Systems

Respiratory System

The Senses

Urinary System

away from, cessation, without

Word Building Example:

dealbation
(de-alb-ation)

The act of whitening, bleaching, or blanching.

---

two, twice

Word Building Example:

disaccharide
(di-sacchar-ide)

A condensation product of two monosaccharides by elimination of water.

---

in two, apart, not

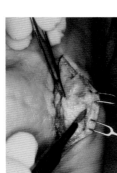

Word Building Example:

dissect
(dis-sect)

1. To cut apart or separate the tissues of the body for study. 2. In an operation, to separate the different structures along natural lines by dividing the connective tissue framework.

---

opposite, opposed, against

Word Building Example:

counterirritation
(counter-irritation)

Irritation or mild inflammation (redness, vesication, or pustulation) of the skin excited for the purpose of relieving symptoms of an inflammation of the deeper structures.

---

one-tenth

Word Building Example:

decimeter
(deci-meter)

One tenth of a meter.

---

through, throughout, completely

Word Building Example:

diameter
(dia-meter)

A straight line connecting two opposite points on the surface of a more or less spherical or cylindrical body, or at the boundary of an opening or foramen, passing through the center of such body or opening.

dys-

Prefix

General Terminology

Prefix

Combining Form

Suffix

e-, ec-, ecto-

General Terminology

Prefix

echo-

Prefix

General Terminology
Cardiovascular System

Prefix

Blood and the Immune System

Cardiovascular System

Endocrine System

Gastrointestinal System

General Terminology

Integumentary System

en-, endo-, em-, ento-

General Terminology

Prefix

epi-

Prefix

General Terminology

Prefix

Musculoskeletal System

Nervous System and Mental Health

Reproductive Systems

Respiratory System

The Senses

Urinary System

equi-

General Terminology

Prefix

out, away from, on the outside

ectopic pregnancy
(ec-top-ic) pregnancy

Implantation and development of a blastocyst outside the uterine cavity.

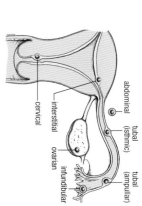

abdominal

interstitial

cervical

tubal (isthmic)

ovarian

tubal (ampullar)

infundibular

---

within, inner, absorbing, containing

endaural
(end-aur-al)

Within the ear.

---

equal, same

equitoxic
(equi-tox-ic)

Of equivalent toxicity.

---

bad, difficult, opposite of eu-

dyshidrosis
(dys-hidr-osis)

A vesicular or vesicopustular eruption of multiple causes that occurs primarily on the volar surfaces of the hands and feet; the lesions spread peripherally but have a tendency to central clearing.

---

a reverberating sound, acoustic signal on ultrasonography

echocardiography
(echo-cardio-graphy)

The use of ultrasound in the investigation of the structure and motion of the heart and great vessels and diagnosis of cardiovascular lesions.

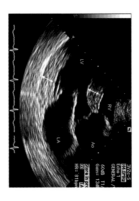

---

upon, following, or subsequent to

epidermis
(epi-derm-is)

1. Superficial epithelial portion of the skin (cutis). 2. In botany, the outermost layer of cells in leaves and the young parts of plants.

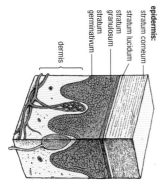

epidermis:

stratum corneum

stratum lucidum

stratum granulosum

stratum germinativum

dermis

eu-

Endocrine System

exo-

General Terminology

Prefix

hemi-

General Terminology

Prefix

eso-

General Terminology

Prefix

- Prefix
- Combining Form
- Suffix

ex-

General Terminology

Prefix

- Blood and the Immune System
- Cardiovascular System
- Endocrine System
- Gastrointestinal System
- General Terminology
- Integumentary System

extra-

General Terminology

Prefix

- Musculoskeletal System
- Nervous System and Mental Health
- Reproductive Systems
- Respiratory System
- The Senses
- Urinary System

good, well; opposite of dys-

Word Building Example:

eugenics
(eu-gen-ics)

Practices and policies, as of mate selection or of sterilization, which tend to better the innate qualities of progeny and human stock.

---

inward

Word Building Example:

esotropia
(eso-tropia)

The form of strabismus in which the visual axes converge; may be paralytic or concomitant, monocular or alternating, accommodative or nonaccommodative.

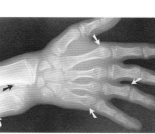

---

exterior, external, outward

Word Building Example:

exostosis
(exo-osto-sis)

A cartilage-capped bony projection arising from any bone that develops from cartilage.

arrows show several small osteochondromas

---

out of, from, away from

Word Building Example:

exophthalmos
(ex-opthalm-os)

Protrusion of one or both eyeballs; can be congenital and familial, or due to pathology, such as a retroorbital tumor (usually unilateral) or thyroid disease (usually bilateral).

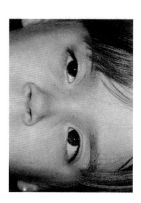

---

one-half

Word Building Example:

hemialgia
(hemi-algia)

Pain affecting one entire half of the body.

---

without, outside of

Word Building Example:

extrasensory
(extra-sensory)

Outside or beyond the ordinary senses; not limited to the senses, as in extrasensory perception.

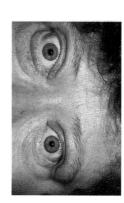

Cardiovascular System

holo-

General Terminology

hetero-

Prefix

Combining Form

Suffix

General Terminology

hyper-

Prefix

General Terminology

homo-, homeo-

Prefix

Blood and the Immune System

Cardiovascular System

Endocrine System

Gastrointestinal System

General Terminology

Integumentary System

General Terminology

im-

Prefix

General Terminology

Nervous System and Mental Health

hypo-

Prefix

Musculoskeletal System

Nervous System and Mental Health

Reproductive Systems

Respiratory System

The Senses

Urinary System

whole, entire, complete

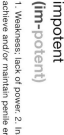

Word Building Example:

holoacardius
(holo-a-cardi-us)

A separate, grossly defective twin lacking a heart of its own, its blood supply being dependent on a shunt from the placental circulation of a more nearly normal twin.

---

excessive, above normal; opposite of hypo-

An ocular condition in which only convergent rays can be brought to focus on the retina.

Word Building Example:

hyperopia
(hyper-opia)

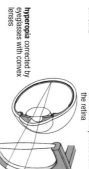

normal (20/20) vision, light rays focus sharply on retina

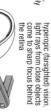

hyperopic (farsighted) vision, light rays from close objects come to sharp focus behind the retina

hyperopia corrected by eyeglasses with convex lenses

---

not

Word Building Example:

impotent
(im-potent)

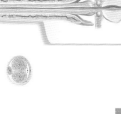

1. Weakness; lack of power. 2. Inability of the male to achieve and/or maintain penile erection and thus engage in copulation.

---

the other, different; opposite of homo-

Surgical division of the constriction or strangulation of a hernia, often followed by herniorrhaphy.

Word Building Example:

heteroduplex
(hetero-duplex)

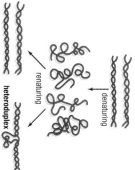

heteroduplex

renaturing

denaturing

---

the same, alike

The state of equilibrium (balance between opposing pressures) in the body with respect to various functions and to the chemical compositions of the fluids and tissues.

Word Building Example:

homeostasis
(homeo-stasis)

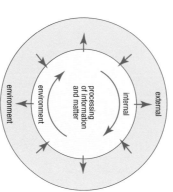

processing of information and matter

internal

external

environment

environment

---

deficient, below normal, under, less than

A condition of having less than the normal complement of teeth, either congenital or acquired.

Word Building Example:

hypodontia
(hypo-dont-ia)

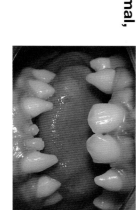

infra-

General Terminology

in-

General Terminology

Prefix

Combining Form

Suffix

intra-

Prefix

General Terminology

inter-

General Terminology

Prefix

Blood and the Immune System

Cardiovascular System

Endocrine System

Gastrointestinal System

General Terminology

Integumentary System

ipsi-

Prefix

General Terminology

intro-

General Terminology

Prefix

Musculoskeletal System

Nervous System and Mental Health

Reproductive Systems

Respiratory System

The Senses

Urinary System

below, beneath, or under

Word Building Example:
**infracardiac
(infra-cardi-ac)**
Beneath the heart; below the level of the heart.

**not
in, within, inside**

**inside, within;
opposite of extra-**

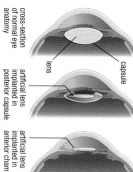

cross-section
of normal eye
anatomy

capsule

lens

artificial lens
implanted in
posterior capsule

artificial lens
implanted in
anterior chamber

Word Building Example:
**intraocular implant
(intra-ocul-ar) implant**
A plastic lens placed in the anterior or posterior chamber of the eye to substitute for the lens removed in cataract extraction.

---

same

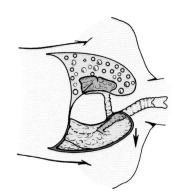

Word Building Example:
**ipsilateral
(ipsi-later-al)**
On the same side, with reference to a given point, e.g., a dilated pupil on the same side as an extradural hematoma.

Word Building Example:
**inhalation
(in-hal-ation)**
1. The act of drawing in the breath. 2. Drawing a medicated vapor in with the breath. 3. A solution of a drug or combination of drugs for administration as a nebulized mist intended to reach the respiratory tree.

---

among, between

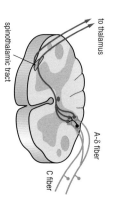

to thalamus

spinothalamic tract

A-δ fiber

C fiber

Word Building Example:
**interneurons
(inter-neurons)**
Combinations or groups of neurons between sensory and motor neurons that govern coordinated activity.

**inwardly, into;
opposite of extra-**

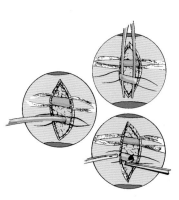

Word Building Example:
**introgastric
(intro-gastr-ic)**
Leading or passed into the stomach.

juxta-

General Terminology

iso-

General Terminology

Prefix
Combining Form
Suffix

macro-

Prefix

General Terminology

kilo-

Prefix

General Terminology

Blood and the Immune System
Cardiovascular System
Endocrine System
Gastrointestinal System
General Terminology
Integumentary System

medio-

Prefix

General Terminology

mal-

Prefix

General Terminology

Musculoskeletal System
Nervous System and Mental Health
Reproductive Systems
Respiratory System
The Senses
Urinary System

near to, beside

Word Building Example:

juxtaglomerular apparatus
(**juxta-glomerul-ar**) apparatus

A complex consisting of the juxtaglomerular cells, which are modified smooth muscle cells in the wall of the afferent glomerular arteriole and sometimes also the efferent arteriole

---

large, long

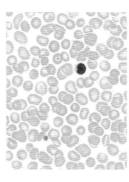

---

equal, alike, sameness

Word Building Example:

isobaric
(**iso-bar-ic**)

1. Having equal weights or pressures. 2. With respect to solutions, having the same density as the diluent or medium; e.g., in spinal anesthesia, an isobaric solution has the same specific gravity as spinal fluid.

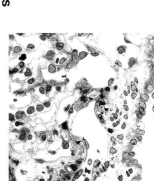
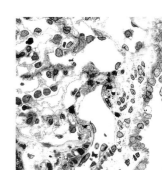

Word Building Example:

macrocythemia
(**macro-cyt-hemia**)

The occurrence of unusually large numbers of macrocytes in the circulating blood.

middle, median

Word Building Example:

medionecrosis
(**medio-necr-osis**)

Necrosis of tunica media.

Word Building Example:

kilogram
(**kilo-gram**)

The SI unit of mass, 1000 g.

one thousand

---

ill, bad; opposite of eu-

Word Building Example:

malabsorption
(**mal-absorption**)

Imperfect, inadequate, or otherwise disordered gastrointestinal absorption.

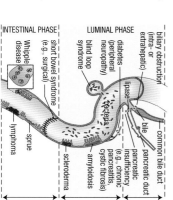

meso-

General Terminology

micro-

General Terminology

Prefix

mio-

General Terminology

Prefix

mega-, megalo-

General Terminology

Prefix

Combining Form

Suffix

meta-

General Terminology

Prefix

Blood and the Immune System

Cardiovascular System

Endocrine System

Gastrointestinal System

General Terminology

Integumentary System

milli-

General Terminology

Prefix

Musculoskeletal System

Nervous System and Mental Health

Reproductive Systems

Respiratory System

The Senses

Urinary System

middle, mean, intermediacy
mesentery or mesentery-like
structure

Word Building Example:

**mesorrhaphy
(meso-rraphy)**

Any product or substrate of metabolism, especially of catabolism.

small

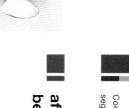

large, abnormally large

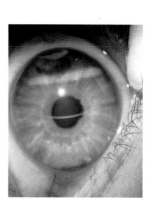

Word Building Example:

**megalocornea
(megalo-cornea)**

Congenital anomaly consisting of an enlarged anterior segment of the eye.

after, subsequent to,
behind, or hindmost

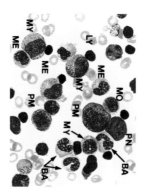

Word Building Example:

**metamyelocyte
(meta-myelo-cyte)**

A transitional form of myelocyte with nuclear construction intermediate between the mature myelocyte and the two-lobed granular leukocyte.

less, smaller

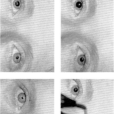

Word Building Example:

**microdontia
(micro-don't-ia)**

A condition in which a single tooth, or pairs of teeth, or the whole dentition, is disproportionately small.

one-thousandth

Word Building Example:

**millimeter
(milli-meter)**

One thousandth of a meter.

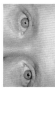

**miosis
(mio-sis)**

Contraction of the pupil.

multi-

General Terminology

Prefix

mono-

General Terminology

Prefix

Combining Form

Suffix

Prefix

neo-

General Terminology

Prefix

nano-

General Terminology

Blood and the Immune System

Cardiovascular System

Endocrine System

Gastrointestinal System

General Terminology

Integumentary System

Prefix

non-

General Terminology

Prefix

noci-

General Terminology

Musculoskeletal System

Nervous System and Mental Health

Reproductive Systems

Respiratory System

The Senses

Urinary System

Word Building Example:

**multicellular
(multi-cellul-ar)**

Composed of many cells.

Word Building Example:

**neonatal
(neo-nat-al)**

Relating to the period immediately after birth through
the first 28 days of life.

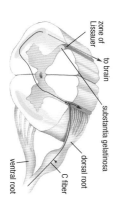

Word Building Example:

**nonproteogenic
(non-proteo-genic)**

Not leading to the production of proteins.

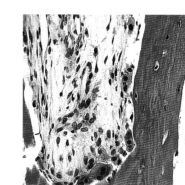

Word Building Example:

**monozygotic twins
(mono-zygo-tic) twins**

Twins resulting from a single zygote
that at an early stage of development
separate into independently growing cell
aggregations creating two individuals
of the same sex and identical genetic
constitution.

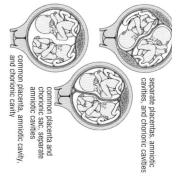

separate placentas, amniotic
cavities, and chorionic cavities

common placenta and
chorionic sac, separate
amniotic cavities

common placenta, amniotic cavity,
and chorionic cavity

Word Building Example:

**nanogram
(nano-gram)**

One billionth of a gram (10^{-9} g).

Word Building Example:

**nociceptive
(noci-ceptive)**

Capable of appreciation or transmission of pain.

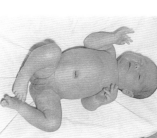

zone of
Lissauer

to brain

substantia gelatinosa

dorsal root

C fiber

ventral root

Card 74

nulli-

General Terminology

Card 76

oo-

Reproductive Systems

Prefix

Card 78

pachy-

General Terminology

Prefix

Card 73

normo-

General Terminology

Prefix

Prefix

Combining Form

Suffix

Card 75

octa-, octi-, octo-

General Terminology

Prefix

Blood and the Immune System

Cardiovascular System

Endocrine System

Gastrointestinal System

General Terminology

Integumentary System

Card 77

oxy-

General Terminology

Prefix

Musculoskeletal System

Nervous System and Mental Health

Reproductive Systems

Respiratory System

The Senses

Urinary System

ovum

Word Building Example:

nulligravida
(nulli-gravid-a)

A woman who has never conceived a child.

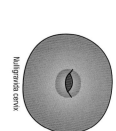

Nulligravida cervix

Word Building Example:

oogonium
(oo-gon-ium)

Primordial germ cells. In fungi, female gametangium bearing one or more oospores.

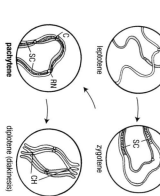

1st trimester

oogonium

mitosis

oogonium
(46 chromosomes)

oogonium

thick

Word Building Example:

pachytene
(pachy-tene)

The stage of prophase in meiosis in which pairing of homologous chromosomes is complete and the paired homologues may twine about each other as they continue to shorten.

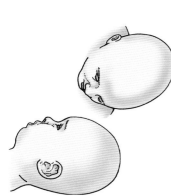

leptotene

zygotene

SC

C
SC
RN

pachytene

diplotene (diakinesis)

CH

Word Building Example:

normocyte
(normo-cyte)

A red blood cell of normal size, shape, and color.

eight

**octose
(octa-ose)**

A sugar containing eight carbon atoms.

eshrill, sharp, pointed, quick/denoting the presence of oxygen

Word Building Example:

oxycephaly
(oxy-cephal-y)

A type of craniosynostosis in which there is premature closure of the lambdoid and coronal sutures, resulting in an abnormally high, peaked, or cone-shaped cranium.

para-

per-

polio-

Nervous System & Mental Health

General Terminology

Prefix

General Terminology

Prefix

Nervous System & Mental Health

Prefix

pan-

penta-

peri-

General Terminology

Prefix

General Terminology

Prefix

General Terminology

Prefix

Prefix

Combining Form

Suffix

Blood and the Immune System

Cardiovascular System

Endocrine System

Gastrointestinal System

General Terminology

Integumentary System

Musculoskeletal System

Nervous System and Mental Health

Reproductive Systems

Respiratory System

The Senses

Urinary System

adjacent, beside, near

departure from the normal

Word Building Example:

paranasal sinuses (para-nas-al) sinuses

Paired air-filled cavities in facial bones lined by mucous membrane continuous with that of the nasal cavity.

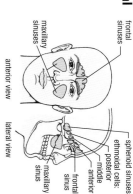

frontal sinuses
maxillary sinuses
anterior view
sphenoid sinuses
ethmoidal cells:
— posterior
— middle
— anterior
frontal sinus
maxillary sinus
lateral view

through, conveying intensity

Word Building Example:

perforation (per-foration)

Abnormal opening in a hollow organ or viscus.

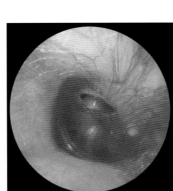

gray, gray matter

Word Building Example:

poliomyelitis (polio-myel-itis)

An inflammatory process involving the gray matter of the spinal cord.

---

all, entire

Word Building Example:

panangiitis (pan-angi-itis)

Inflammation of all layers of a blood vessel.

five

Word Building Example:

pentapeptide (penta-peptide)

A compound containing five amino acyl residues linked via peptide bonds.

around, about, near

Word Building Example:

perichondritis (peri-chrondr-itis)

Inflammation of the dense irregular connective tissue membrane around cartilage.

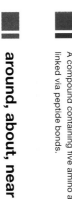

Card 85

poly-

General Terminology

- **Prefix**
- **Combining Form**
- **Suffix**

Card 86

post-

General Terminology

Card 87

pre-

General Terminology

Prefix

- Blood and the Immune System
- Cardiovascular System
- Endocrine System
- **Gastrointestinal System**
- General Terminology
- Integumentary System

Card 88

primi-

Prefix

Reproductive Systems

Card 89

pro-

General Terminology

Prefix

- Musculoskeletal System
- Nervous System and Mental Health
- Reproductive Systems
- **Respiratory System**
- The Senses
- Urinary System

Card 90

pseudo-

Prefix

after, behind, posterior; opposite of anti-

Word Building Example:
postclavicular
(**post-clavicul-ar**)

Posterior to the clavicle.

---

first, one

---

false (often used about a deceptive resemblance)

Word Building Example:
primigravida
(**primi-gravida**)

A woman who is pregnant for the first time.

Word Building Example:
pseudoisochromatic
(**pseudo-iso-chromat-ic**)

Apparently of the same color; denoting certain charts containing colored spots mixed with figures printed in confusing colors; used in testing for color vision deficiency.

---

many, multiplicity

Word Building Example:
polychromatophilic
(**poly-chromato-phil-ic**)

Having a tendency to stain with both basic and acidic dyes.

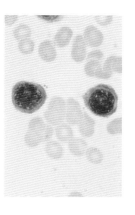

---

anterior

before (in time or space)

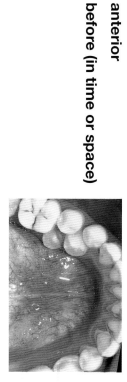

Word Building Example:
premolar
(**pre-molar**)

Anterior to a molar tooth.

---

before, forward

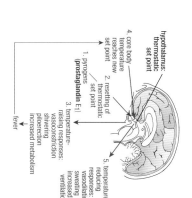

Word Building Example:
prodrome
(**pro-drome**)

An early or premonitory symptom of a disease.

puer-

Reproductive Systems

ptyal-, ptyalo-

The Senses

Prefix

Combining Form

Suffix

re-

General Terminology

Prefix

quadri-

General Terminology

Prefix

Blood and the Immune System

Cardiovascular System

Endocrine System

Gastrointestinal System

General Terminology

Integumentary System

semi-

General Terminology

Prefix

retro-

General Terminology

Prefix

Musculoskeletal System

Nervous System and Mental Health

Reproductive Systems

Respiratory System

The Senses

Urinary System

child

Word Building Example:

**puerperium
(puer-peri-um)**

Period from the termination of labor to complete involution of the uterus, usually defined as 42 days.

---

backward, again

Word Building Example:

**ptyalocele
(ptyalo-cele)**

Any cystic tumor of the undersurface of the tongue or floor of the mouth, especially one of the floor of the mouth due to obstruction of the duct of the sublingual glands.

Word Building Example:

**rehabilitation
(re-habil-itation)**

Spontaneous or therapeutic restoration, after disease, illness, or injury, of the ability to function in a normal or near normal manner.

---

one-half, partly

---

four

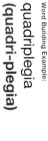

monoplegia

tetraplegia or
quadriplegia

hemiplegia

paraplegia

---

salivary glands, saliva

Word Building Example:

**semicomatose
(semi-coma-tose)**

An imprecise term for a state of drowsiness and inaction, in which more than ordinary stimulation may be required to evoke a response, and the response may be delayed or

---

Word Building Example:

**quadriplegia
(quadri-plegia)**

Paralysis of all four limbs.

---

backward, behind

Word Building Example:

**retrovirus
(retro-virus)**

Any virus of the family Retroviridae. A virus with RNA core genetic material; requires the enzyme reverse transcriptase to convert its RNA into proviral DNA.

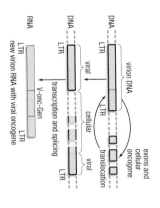

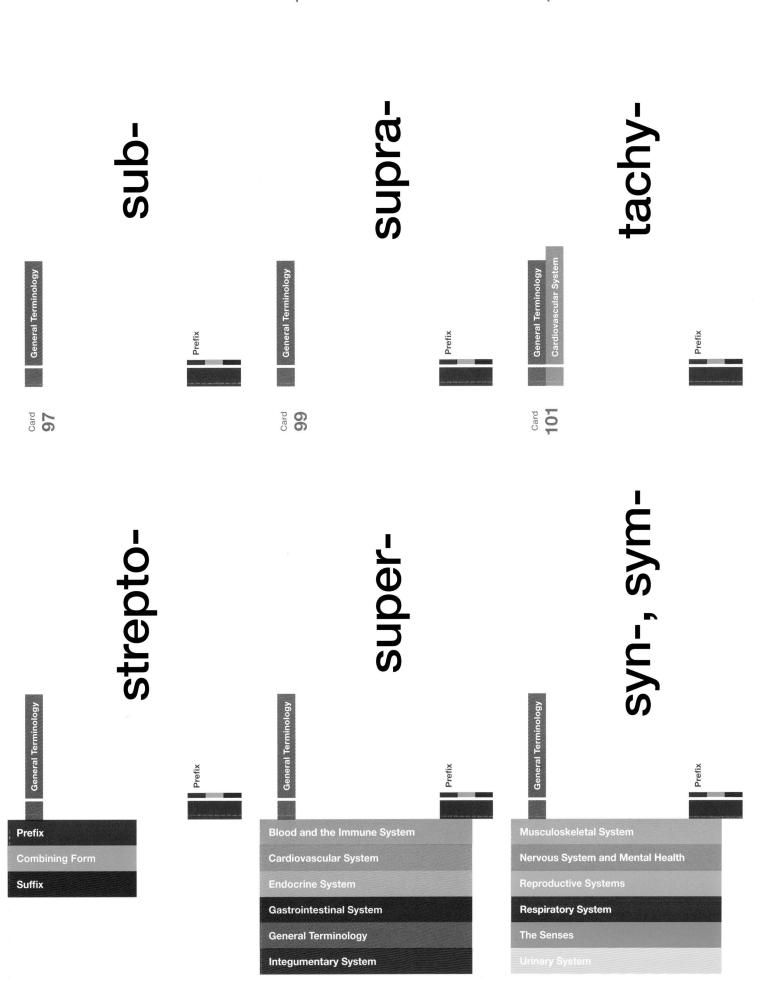

Card
97

Card
98

sub-

General Terminology

Prefix

Card
99

Card
100

supra-

General Terminology

Prefix

Card
101

Card
102

tachy-

General Terminology

Cardiovascular System

Prefix

strepto-

General Terminology

Prefix
Combining Form
Suffix

Prefix

super-

General Terminology

Blood and the Immune System
Cardiovascular System
Endocrine System
Gastrointestinal System
General Terminology
Integumentary System

Prefix

syn-, sym-

General Terminology

Musculoskeletal System
Nervous System and Mental Health
Reproductive Systems
Respiratory System
The Senses
Urinary System

Prefix

beneath, less than the normal or typical, inferior

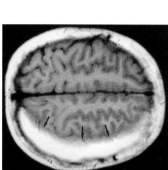

Word Building Example:
subdural
(sub-dur-al)

1. Deep to the dura mater. 2. Between the dura mater and the arachnoid mater.

---

curved or twisted (usually referring to organisms)

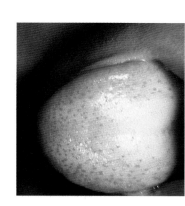

Word Building Example:
streptococcal
(strepto-cocc-al)

Relating to or caused by any organism of the genus Streptococcus.

---

a position above the part indicated by the word to which it is joined; in this sense, the same as super-; opposite of infra-

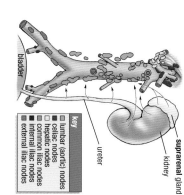

bladder

ureter

suprarenal gland

kidney

key
- lumbar (aortic) nodes
- celiac nodes
- hepatic nodes
- common iliac nodes
- internal iliac nodes
- external iliac nodes

Word Building Example:
suprarenal
(supra-ren-al)

1. Above the kidney. 2. Pertaining to the suprarenal glands.

---

rapid

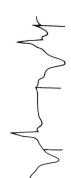

Word Building Example:
tachycardia
(tachy-cardi-a)

Rapid beating of the heart, conventionally applied to rates over 90 beats per minute.

---

in excess, above, superior, or in the upper part of; often the same usage as supra- or hyper-

Word Building Example:
supramarginal
(supra-margin-al)

Above any margin.

---

together, with, joined

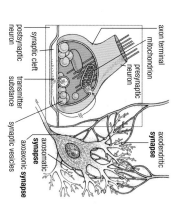

axon terminal
mitochondrion

synaptic cleft

postsynaptic
neuron

presynaptic
neuron

transmitter
substance

synaptic vesicles

axodendritic
synapse

axosomatic
synapse

axoaxonic **synapse**

Word Building Example:
synapse
(syn-apse)

The functional membrane-to-membrane contact of the nerve cell with another nerve cell, an effector (muscle, gland) cell, or a sensory receptor cell.

tetra-

General Terminology

tri-

Prefix

General Terminology

un-

Prefix

General Terminology

Prefix

Prefix

tele-, telo-

General Terminology

Prefix

Combining Form

Suffix

trans-

General Terminology

Prefix

Blood and the Immune System

Cardiovascular System

Endocrine System

Gastrointestinal System

General Terminology

Integumentary System

ultra-

General Terminology

Prefix

Musculoskeletal System

Nervous System and Mental Health

Reproductive Systems

Respiratory System

The Senses

Urinary System

four

Word Building Example:

tetracycline
(tetra-cycl-ine)

A broad spectrum antibiotic (a naphthacene derivative), the parent of oxytetracycline, prepared from chlortetracycline and also obtained from the culture filtrate of several species of *Streptomyces*. Tetracycline fluorescence has been used in studies of growing tumors and calcium deposition in developing bones and teeth.

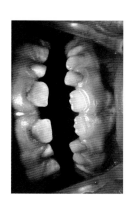

distance, end, other end

Word Building Example:

telophase
(telo-phase)

The final stage of mitosis or meiosis, which begins when migration of chromosomes to the poles of the cell has been completed.

nucleolus
nucleus
prophase
centriole

anaphase

metaphase
spindle
fibers

telophase

---

three

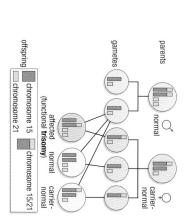

parents

normal

carrier-normal

gametes

affected
(functional **trisomy**)
normal
normal
carrier-normal

offspring

chromosome 15
chromosome 21
chromosome 15/21

across, through, beyond

Word Building Example:

transcription
(trans-script-ion)

1. Transfer of genetic code information from one kind of nucleic acid to another. 2. Process in which medical transcriptionists convert dictated health care information into a printed document.

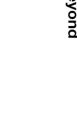

promoter
transcription unit
terminator

RNA polymerase

P–P–P–N
P–P–P–A
or
P–P–P–G
binding
initiation

growing RNA
(nlP–P–P–N)
elongation

completed RNA
P–P–P–A–N–N–N–N–N–N–N–N–N–N–N–N–N–N–OH
termination

---

not

Word Building Example:

trisomy
(tri-somy)

The state of an individual or cell with an extra chromosome instead of the normal pair of homologous chromosomes.

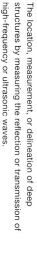
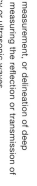

excess, exaggeration, beyond

Word Building Example:

ultrasonography
(ultra-sono-graphy)

The location, measurement, or delineation of deep structures by measuring the reflection or transmission of high-frequency or ultrasonic waves.

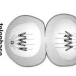

transducer
skin
sound waves
internal organ
principle of sonography

---

unconscious
(un-con-scious)

Lacking awareness.

xeno-

General Terminology

uni-

General Terminology

Prefix

Combining Form

Suffix

-ac

Prefix

General Terminology

Suffix

xero-

Integumentary System

The Senses

Prefix

Blood and the Immune System

Cardiovascular System

Endocrine System

Gastrointestinal System

General Terminology

Integumentary System

-ad

General Terminology

Suffix

-acusis, -cusis

The Senses

Suffix

Musculoskeletal System

Nervous System and Mental Health

Reproductive Systems

Respiratory System

The Senses

Urinary System

foreign, strange

Word Building Example:

xenobiotic
(xeno-bio-tic)

A pharmacologically, endocrinologically, or toxicologically active substance not endogenously produced and therefore foreign to an organism.

---

pertaining to, relating to

---

toward

Word Building Example:

cardiac
(cardi-ac)

Pertaining to the heart.

Word Building Example:

triad
(tri-ad)

A group of three things with something in common.

---

one, single, not paired

Word Building Example:

unilateral
(uni-later-al)

Confined to one side only.

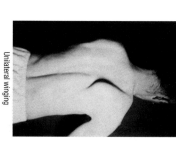

Unilateral winging

---

dry

Word Building Example:

xeroderma
(xero-derma)

A mild form of ichthyosis characterized by excessive dryness of the skin due to slight thickening of the horny layer and diminished water content of the stratum corneum from decreased perspiration or exposure to wind, or low humidity; seen with aging, atopic dermatitis, and vitamin A deficiency.

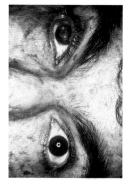

---

hearing condition

Word Building Example:

presbyacusis
(presby-acusis)

Loss of hearing associated with aging; manifest as reduced ability to perceive or discriminate sounds; the pattern and age of onset vary.

-al

General Terminology

Suffix

-agra

General Terminology

Suffix

Prefix

Combining Form

Suffix

-ar

General Terminology

Suffix

-algia, -algesia

General Terminology

Suffix

Blood and the Immune System

Cardiovascular System

Endocrine System

Gastrointestinal System

General Terminology

Integumentary System

-arthria

The Senses

Suffix

-arche

Reproductive Systems

Suffix

Musculoskeletal System

Nervous System and Mental Health

Reproductive Systems

Respiratory System

The Senses

Urinary System

pertaining to, relating to

Word Building Example:

abaxial
(ab-axi-al)

1. Lying outside the axis of any body or part. 2. Situated at the opposite extremity of the axis of a part.

pertaining to, relating to

muscular
(muscul-ar)

Relating to a muscle or the muscles.

Word Building Example:

articulate

dysarthria
(dys-arthria)

A disturbance of speech due to paralysis, incoordination, or spasticity of the muscles used for speaking.

Word Building Example:

sudden onslaught of
acute pain

Word Building Example:

podagra
(podo-agra)

Severe pain in the foot, especially that of typical gout in the great toe.

pain

fibromyalgia
(fibro-my-algia)

A condition involving lack of stage IV sleep and chronic diffuse widespread aching and stiffness of muscles and soft tissues.

Word Building Example:

beginning

menarche
(men-arche)

Establishment of the menstrual function; the time of the first menstrual period.

Word Building Example:

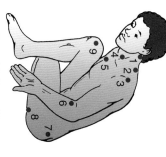

Fibromyalgia trigger points

-ase

General Terminology

Suffix

-ary

General Terminology

Suffix

Prefix

Combining Form

Suffix

-ate

General Terminology

Suffix

-asthenia

Musculoskeletal System

Suffix

Blood and the Immune System

Cardiovascular System

Endocrine System

Gastrointestinal System

General Terminology

Integumentary System

-capnia

Respiratory System

Suffix

-blast

General Terminology

Suffix

Musculoskeletal System

Nervous System and Mental Health

Reproductive Systems

Respiratory System

The Senses

Urinary System

enzyme

lactase
(lact-ase)

Word Building Example:

A sugar-splitting enzyme that catalyzes the hydrolysis of lactose into D-glucose and D-galactose, and that of other β-D-galactosides

---

a salt or ester of an acid ending with "-ic"

carbonate
(carbon-ate)

Word Building Example:

A salt of carbonic acid.

carbon dioxide

---

normocapnia
(normo-capnia)

Word Building Example:

A state in which the arterial carbon dioxide pressure is normal, about 40 mmHg.

---

pertaining to, relating to

maxillary artery
(maxill-ary) artery

Word Building Example:

Origin, external carotid; branches, deep auricular, anterior tympanic, middle meningeal, inferior alveolar, masseteric, deep temporal, buccal, posterior superior alveolar, infraorbital, descending palatine, artery of pterygoid canal, sphenopalatine.

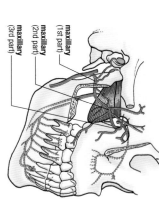

maxillary (1st part)
maxillary (2nd part)
maxillary (3rd part)

weakness

---

thrombocytasthenia
(thrombo-asthenia)

Word Building Example:

A term for a group of hemorrhagic disorders in which the platelets may be only slightly reduced in number, or even within the normal range, but are morphologically abnormal, or are lacking in factors that are effective in the coagulation of blood.

immature precursor cell type

---

sideroblast
(sidero-blast)

Word Building Example:

An erythroblast containing granules of ferritin stained by the Prussian blue reaction.

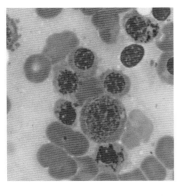

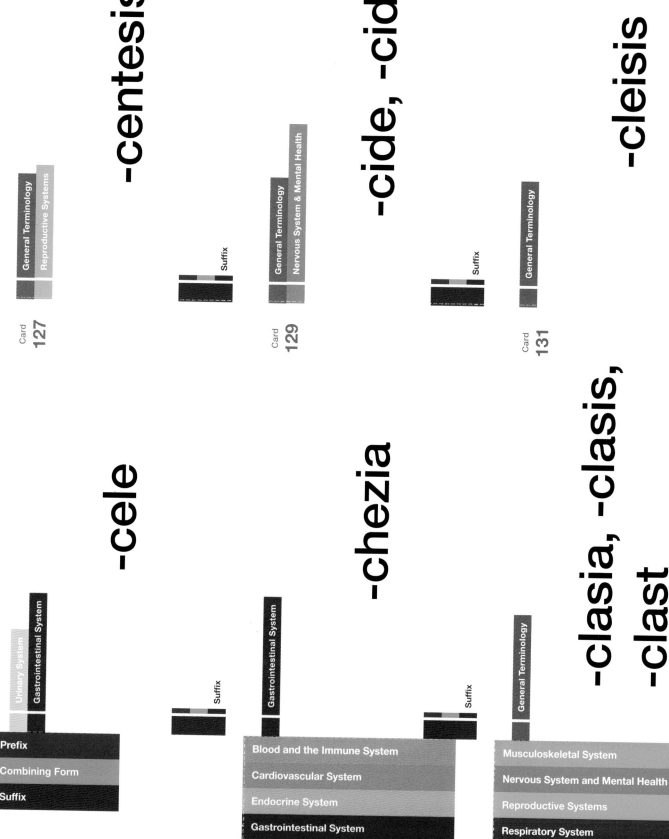

Card 128 — -centesis

Card 127 — General Terminology / Reproductive Systems — Suffix

Card 130 — -cide, -cidal

Card 129 — General Terminology / Nervous System & Mental Health — Suffix

Card 132 — -cleisis

Card 131 — General Terminology — Suffix

-cele

Urinary System / Gastrointestinal System

Prefix
Combining Form
Suffix

-chezia

Gastrointestinal System — Suffix

Blood and the Immune System
Cardiovascular System
Endocrine System
Gastrointestinal System
General Terminology
Integumentary System

-clasia, -clasis, -clast

General Terminology — Suffix

Musculoskeletal System
Nervous System and Mental Health
Reproductive Systems
Respiratory System
The Senses
Urinary System

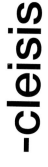
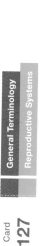

puncture, tap

Word Building Example:

amniocentesis
(amnio-centesis)

Transabdominal aspiration of fluid from the amniotic sac for diagnostic purposes.

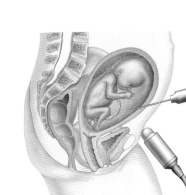
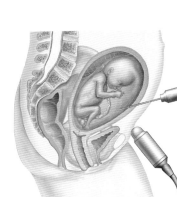

agent that kills, or act of killing

Word Building Example:

bactericide
(bacteri-cide)

An agent that destroys bacteria.

closure

Word Building Example:

hysterocleisis
(hystero-cleisis)

Operative occlusion of the uterus.

hernia, swelling

Word Building Example:

gastrocele
(gastro-cele)

Hernia of part of the stomach.

defecation

Word Building Example:

dyschezia
(dys-chezia)

Difficulty in defecation.

break, breaking

Word Building Example:

osteoclast
(osteo-clast)

A large multinucleated cell, possibly of monocytic origin, with abundant acidophilic cytoplasm, functioning in the absorption and removal of osseous tissue.

-coccus

General Terminology

Suffix

-crine

Endocrine System

Suffix

-cyte, cyt/o

General Terminology

Suffix

-clysis

General Terminology

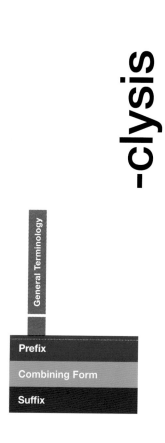

Prefix

Combining Form

Suffix

Suffix

-crasia

General Terminology

Blood and the Immune System

Blood and the Immune System

Cardiovascular System

Endocrine System

Gastrointestinal System

General Terminology

Integumentary System

Suffix

-cyesis

Reproductive Systems

Musculoskeletal System

Nervous System and Mental Health

Reproductive Systems

Respiratory System

The Senses

Urinary System

Suffix

berry-shaped bacterium

infusion of fluid, injection, enema

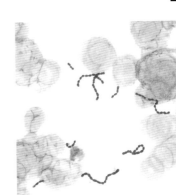

Word Building Example:

streptococcus
(strepto-**coccus**)

A term used to refer to any member of the genus *Streptococcus*.

Word Building Example:

enteroclysis
(entero-**clysis**)

An enema instilled high up into the colon.

to secrete

mixture or bleeding

Word Building Example:

exocrine
(**exo**-crine)

1. Denoting grandular secretion delivered onto the body surface. 2. Denoting a gland that secretes outwardly through excretory ducts.

Word Building Example:

galactacrasia
(galacta-**crasia**)

Abnormal composition of mother's milk.

cell

pregnancy

Word Building Example:

cytogenetics
(cyto-gene-**tics**)

The branch of genetics concerned with the structure and function of the cell, especially the chromosomes.

Word Building Example:

oocyesis
(oo-**cyesis**)

Development of an impregnated oocyte in an ovarian follicle.

-desis

Musculoskeletal System

-cytosis

General Terminology

Suffix

Prefix

Combining Form

Suffix

-dote

General Terminology

Suffix

-dilation, -dilatation

General Terminology

Suffix

Blood and the Immune System

Cardiovascular System

Endocrine System

Gastrointestinal System

General Terminology

Integumentary System

-dynia

General Terminology

Suffix

Suffix

-drome

General Terminology

Suffix

Musculoskeletal System

Nervous System and Mental Health

Reproductive Systems

Respiratory System

The Senses

Urinary System

binding, stabilizing, fixation of a bone or joint, tie together

Word Building Example:

spondylosyndesis
(spondylo-syn-desis)

An operative procedure to accomplish bony ankylosis between two or more vertebrae.

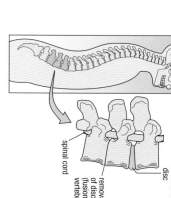

intervertebral disc

removal of disc (fusion of vertebrae)

spinal cord

give

pain

antidote
(anti-dote)

An agent that neutralizes a poison or counteracts its effects.

osteodynia
(osteo-dynia)

Pain in a bone.

---

more than the usual number of cells

Word Building Example:

hypercytosis
(hyper-cytosis)

Any condition with an abnormal increase in the number of cells in the circulating blood or the tissues; frequently used to mean with leukocytosis.

expansion, widening

Word Building Example:

vasodilation
(vaso-dilation)

Increase in the caliber of a blood vessel due to relaxation of smooth muscle fibers in the tunica media. This increases blood flow but decreases systemic vascular resistance.

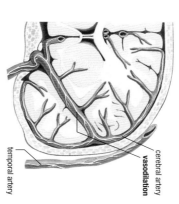

cerebral artery **vasodilation**

temporal artery

running, a course

Word Building Example:

syndrome
(syn-drome)

The combination of signs and symptoms associated with a particular morbid process, which together constitute the picture of a disease or inherited anomaly.

-ectasia, -ectasis

General Terminology
Reproductive Systems

Suffix

-eal, -ile

General Terminology

Suffix

Prefix
Combining Form
Suffix

-edema

General Terminology

Suffix

-ectomy

General Terminology

Suffix

Blood and the Immune System
Cardiovascular System
Endocrine System
Gastrointestinal System
General Terminology
Integumentary System

-emetic

Gastrointestinal System

Suffix

-emesis

Gastrointestinal System

Suffix

Musculoskeletal System
Nervous System and Mental Health
Reproductive Systems
Respiratory System
The Senses
Urinary System

dilation, expansion

Word Building Example:

bronchiectasis
(bronchi-ectasis)

Chronic dilation of bronchi or bronchioles as a sequel of inflammatory disease or obstruction.

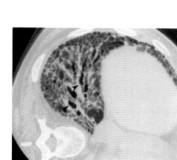

accumulation of fluid, swelling

Word Building Example:

angioedema
(angio-edema)

Recurrent large circumscribed areas of subcutaneous or mucosal edema of sudden onset, usually disappearing within 24 hours; frequently, an allergic reaction to foods or drugs.

pertaining to vomiting

pertaining to

Word Building Example:

meningeal
(mening-eal)

Relating to the meninges.

removal of an anatomical structure

Word Building Example:

vasectomy
(vas-ectomy)

Excision of a segment of the vas deferens, performed in association with prostatectomy, or to produce sterility.

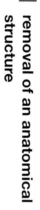

testis

cut and ligated ductus deferens (vas deferens)

seminal vesicle

vomiting

Word Building Example:

antiemetic
(anti-emetic)

Preventing or arresting vomiting.

Word Building Example:

hematemesis
(hemat-emesis)

Vomiting of blood.

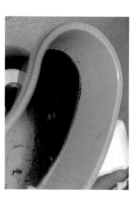

-emia

Blood and the Immune System

Suffix

Prefix

Combining Form

Suffix

-emphraxis

Endocrine System

Suffix

-esis

General Terminology

Suffix

Blood and the Immune System

Cardiovascular System

Endocrine System

Gastrointestinal System

General Terminology

Integumentary System

-esthesia

Integumentary System

Suffix

-flexion

Musculoskeletal System

Suffix

Musculoskeletal System

Nervous System and Mental Health

Reproductive Systems

Respiratory System

The Senses

Urinary System

-form

General Terminology

Suffix

obstruction

Word Building Example:

pancreatemphraxis
(pancreat-emphraxis)

Obstruction in the pancreatic duct, causing swelling
of the gland.

perception, feeling

Word Building Example:

anesthesia
(an-esthesia)

Loss of sensation resulting from pharmacologic depression
of nerve function or from neurologic dysfunction.

like, resembling

bending, flexing

Word Building Example:

pyesis
(py-esis)

The formation of pus.

condition, action, or process

Word Building Example:

anemia
(an-emia)

Any condition in which the number of red blood cells
per mm^3, the amount of hemoglobin in 100 mL of blood,
or the volume of packed red blood cells per 100 mL
of blood is less than normal.

condition of the blood

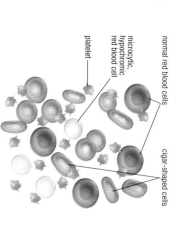

normal red blood cells

microcytic,
hypochromic
red blood cell

platelet

cigar-shaped cells

Word Building Example:

dentiform
(denti-form)

Tooth-shaped; pegged.

Word Building Example:

hyperflexion
(hyper-flexion)

Flexion of a limb or part beyond the normal limit.

-fusion

General Terminology

Suffix

The Senses

-fuge

General Terminology

Suffix

Prefix

Combining Form

Suffix

-geusia

Suffix

-gen, -genesis,
-genic

General Terminology

Suffix

Blood and the Immune System

Cardiovascular System

Endocrine System

Gastrointestinal System

General Terminology

Integumentary System

-grade

General Terminology

Suffix

-globin, -globulin

Blood and the Immune System

Suffix

Musculoskeletal System

Nervous System and Mental Health

Reproductive Systems

Respiratory System

The Senses

Urinary System

pour

transfusion
(trans-fusion)

Transfer of blood or blood component from one person (donor) to another person (receptor).

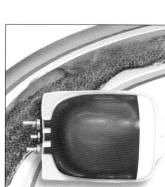

sense of taste

glycogeusia
(glyco-geusia)

A subjective sweet taste.

to step, go step, degree

orthograde
(ortho-grade)

Walking or standing erect; denoting the posture of humans; opposed to pronograde.

to drive away

centrifuge
(centri-fuge)

An apparatus by means of which particles in suspension in a fluid are separated by spinning the fluid, with the centrifugal force throwing the particles to the periphery of the rotated vessel.

precursor of, forming, producing, origin

neurogenic
(neuro-genic)

Originating in, starting from, or caused by, the nervous system or nerve impulses.

name for family of proteins

beta polypeptide chains

iron containing heme

alpha polypeptide chains

O₂

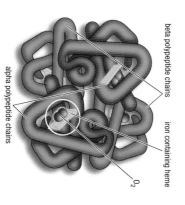

hemoglobin
(hemo-globin)

The red respiratory protein of erythrocytes.

-gram

General Terminology

-graft

General Terminology

Prefix	
Combining Form	
Suffix	

Suffix

-graphy

General Terminology
Cardiovascular System

Suffix

-graph

General Terminology
Cardiovascular System

Suffix

Blood and the Immune System
Cardiovascular System
Endocrine System
Gastrointestinal System
General Terminology
Integumentary System

-ia

General Terminology

Suffix

-gravida

Reproductive Systems

Suffix

Musculoskeletal System
Nervous System and Mental Health
Reproductive Systems
Respiratory System
The Senses
Urinary System

a recording, usually by an instrument

a metric unit of weight

Word Building Example:

sonogram
(sono-gram)

The image obtained by measuring the reflection or transmission of high-frequency or ultrasonic waves.

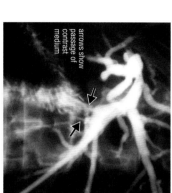

---

a writing or description

Word Building Example:

cholangiography
(chol-angio-graphy)

Radiographic examination of the bile ducts using a contrast medium.

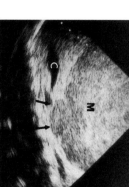

arrows show passage of contrast medium

---

state or condition, often abnormal

Word Building Example:

polyblennia
(poly-blenn-ia)

Excessive production of mucus.

---

transfer

Word Building Example:

autograft
(auto-graft)

A tissue or an organ transferred by grafting into a new position in the body of the same individual.

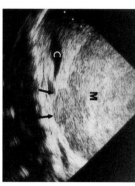

---

line or tracing denoting varying values

instrument used for recording

Word Building Example:

cardiograph
(cardio-graph)

An instrument for recording graphically the movements of the heart, constructed on the principle of the sphygmograph.

---

a pregnant woman

Word Building Example:

multigravida
(multi-gravida)

A pregnant woman who has been pregnant one or more times previously.

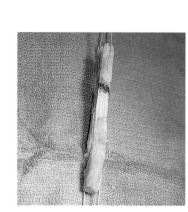

-ian

General Terminology

-iac

General Terminology

- Prefix
- Combining Form
- Suffix

-iatrics, -iatry

General Terminology

Suffix

-iasis

General Terminology

Suffix

- Blood and the Immune System
- Cardiovascular System
- Endocrine System
- Gastrointestinal System
- General Terminology
- Integumentary System

-icle

General Terminology

Suffix

-ic, ical

General Terminology

Suffix

- Musculoskeletal System
- Nervous System and Mental Health
- Reproductive Systems
- Respiratory System
- The Senses
- Urinary System

Word Building Example:

intraovarian
(intra-ovar-ian)

Within the ovary.

---

medical specialty

Word Building Example:

pediatrics
(ped-iatrics)

The medical specialty concerned with the study and treatment of children in health and disease from birth through adolescence.

---

small, little, minute

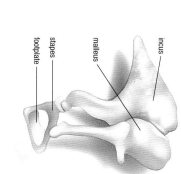

incus
malleus
stapes
footplate

ossicle
(oss-icle)

Word Building Example:

A small bone; specifically, one of the bones of the tympanic cavity or middle ear.

---

achromic
(a-chrom-ic)

Word Building Example:

Colorless.

Word Building Example:

hypochondriac
(hypo-chondr-iac)

1. A person with a somatic overconcern, including morbid attention to the details of bodily functioning and exaggeration of any symptoms no matter how insignificant.
2. Beneath the ribs.

(1) right **hypochondriac**
(2) epigastric
(3) left **hypochondriac**
(4) right lateral (lumbar)
(5) umbilical
(6) left lateral (lumbar)
(7) right iliac
(8) hypogastric (suprapubic)
(9) left iliac

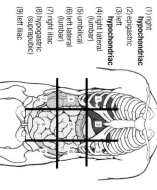

---

condition, infestation, infection (sometimes interchangeable with -osis)

Word Building Example:

broncholithiasis
(broncho-lith-iasis)

Bronchial inflammation or obstruction caused by broncholitits.

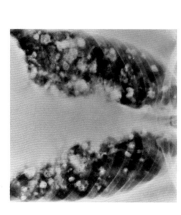

---

pertaining to, relating to

-ictal

Nervous System & Mental Health

Suffix

-ics

General Terminology

Prefix
Combining Form
Suffix

Suffix

-ism

General Terminology

Suffix

-in, -ine

Endocrine System

Blood and the Immune System
Cardiovascular System
Endocrine System
Gastrointestinal System
General Terminology
Integumentary System

Suffix

-ite

Suffix

-ist

General Terminology

Musculoskeletal System
Nervous System and Mental Health
Reproductive Systems
Respiratory System
The Senses
Urinary System

Suffix

stroke, seizure

Word Building Example:

postictal
(post-ictal)

Following a seizure (e.g., epileptic).

---

condition, disease
a practice, doctrine

---

nature of, resembling

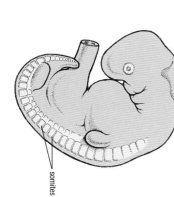

somites

Word Building Example:

somite
(som-ite)

One of the paired, metamerically arranged cell masses
formed in the early embryonic paraxial mesoderm.

Word Building Example:

pleochromatism
(pleo-chromat-ism)

Property of showing changes of color when illuminated
along different axes, as in certain crystals or liquids.

---

medical specialty

Word Building Example:

obstetrics
(obstetr-ics)

The specialty of medicine concerned with the care of
women during pregnancy, parturition, and the puerperium.

---

chemical or biochemical
substance

Word Building Example:

vasopressin
(vaso-press-in)

A nonapeptide neurohypophysial hormone related
to oxytocin and vasotocin. In pharmacologic doses,
vasopressin causes contraction of smooth muscle, notably
that of all blood vessels.

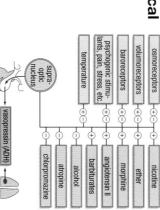

---

specialist

Word Building Example:

somatist
(somat-ist)

An older term for one who considers that neuroses and
psychoses are manifestations of organic disease.

-ium

General Terminology

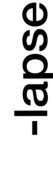

-kinesia, -kinesis

General Terminology

Suffix

-lapse

General Terminology

Suffix

-itis (pl. -itides)

General Terminology

Suffix

Prefix
Combining Form
Suffix

-ization

General Terminology

Suffix

Blood and the Immune System
Cardiovascular System
Endocrine System
Gastrointestinal System
General Terminology
Integumentary System

-lalia

The Senses

Nervous System & Mental Health

Suffix

Musculoskeletal System
Nervous System and Mental Health
Reproductive Systems
Respiratory System
The Senses
Urinary System

Word Building Example:

pericardium
(peri-card-ium)

The fibroserous membrane, consisting of mesothelium and submesothelial connective tissue, covering the heart and beginnings of the great vessels.

movement

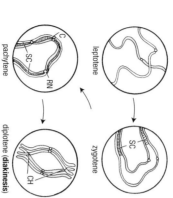

leptotene

zygotene

SC

pachytene

C

SC

RN

diplotene (diakinesis)

CH

Word Building Example:

diakinesis
(dia-kinesis)

Final stage of prophase in meiosis I, in which the chromosomes continue to shorten and the nucleolus and nuclear membrane disappear.

the falling

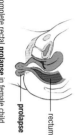

complete rectal **prolapse** in female child

prolapse

rectum

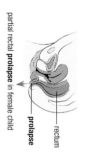

partial rectal **prolapse** in female child

prolapse

rectum

Word Building Example:

prolapse
(pro-lapse)

To sink down; said of an organ or other part.

Word Building Example:

dermatitis
(dermat-itis)

Inflammation of the skin.

the process of

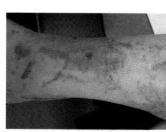

Word Building Example:

pneumatization
(pneumat-ization)

The development of air cells such as those of the mastoid and ethmoidal bones.

speech

Word Building Example:

alalia
(a-lalia)

Mutism; inability to speak.

-lexia

General Terminology
Nervous System & Mental Health

-lepsis, -lepsy

Nervous System & Mental Health

Prefix

Combining Form

Suffix

Suffix

-logist

General Terminology

Suffix

-listhesis

Musculoskeletal System

Suffix

Blood and the Immune System

Cardiovascular System

Endocrine System

Gastrointestinal System

General Terminology

Integumentary System

-lucent

General Terminology

Suffix

-logy, -logia

General Terminology

Suffix

Musculoskeletal System

Nervous System and Mental Health

Reproductive Systems

Respiratory System

The Senses

Urinary System

seizure

Word Building Example:

epilepsy
(epi-lepsy)

A chronic disorder characterized by paroxysmal brain dysfunction due to excessive neuronal discharge; usually associated with some alteration of consciousness; clinical manifestations of the attack may vary from complex abnormalities of behavior including generalized or focal convulsions to momentary spells of impaired consciousness. SYN fit (3), seizure disorder.

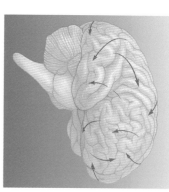

slipping

Word Building Example:

spondylolisthesis
(spondylo-listhesis)

Forward movement of the body of one of the lower lumbar vertebrae on the vertebra below it, or on the sacrum.

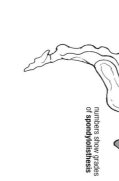

numbers show grades
of **spondylolisthesis**

—L5

study of; collecting or picking

Word Building Example:

radiology
(radio-logy)

Science of high-energy radiation and of the chemical, physical, and biologic effects of such radiation; the term usually refers to the diagnosis and treatment of disease.

Word Building Example:

dyslexia
(dys-lexia)

Impaired reading ability with a competence level below that expected on the basis of the person's level of intelligence, and in the presence of normal vision, letter recognition, and normal recognition of the meaning of pictures and objects.

one who specializes in the study or treatment of

Word Building Example:

pathologist
(patho-logist)

Physician who performs, interprets, or supervises diagnostic tests, using materials removed from living or dead patients, and functions as a laboratory consultant to clinicians, or who conducts experiments or other investigations to determine the causes or nature of disease changes.

to shine

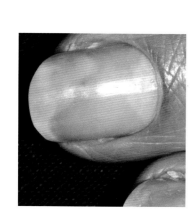

Word Building Example:

translucent
(trans-lucent)

Allowing light to pass through.

-lytic

General Terminology

Suffix

-lysis

General Terminology

Suffix

| Prefix |
| Combining Form |
| Suffix |

-mania

Nervous System & Mental Health

Suffix

-malacia

General Terminology

Suffix

| Blood and the Immune System |
| Cardiovascular System |
| Endocrine System |
| Gastrointestinal System |
| General Terminology |
| Integumentary System |

-meter, -metry

General Terminology

Suffix

-megaly

General Terminology

Suffix

| Musculoskeletal System |
| Nervous System and Mental Health |
| Reproductive Systems |
| Respiratory System |
| The Senses |
| Urinary System |

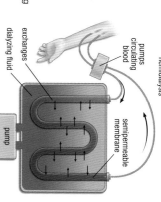
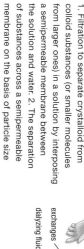

dissolving, reducing, loosening

Word Building Example:

cytolytic
(cyto-lytic)

Pertaining to cytolysis; possessing a solvent or destructive action on cells.

---

abnormal love for, morbid impulse toward

Word Building Example:

megalomania
(megalo-mania)

A type of delusion in which the afflicted person considers himself or herself possessed of greatness.

---

measurement, measurement device

Word Building Example:

radiopelvimetry
(radio-pelvi-metry)

Radiographic measurement of the pelvis.

---

dissolution, loosening

Word Building Example:

dialysis
(dia-lysis)

1. Filtration to separate crystalloid from colloid substances (or smaller molecules from larger ones) in a solution by interposing a semipermeable membrane between the solution and water. 2. The separation of substances across a semipermeable membrane on the basis of particle size and/or concentration gradients. 3. A method of providing artificial kidney function.

hemidialysis

pumps circulating blood

exchanges

dialyzing fluid

semipermeable membrane

pump

---

softening or loss of consistency

Word Building Example:

keratomalacia
(kerato-malacia)

Dryness with ulceration and corneal perforation in cachectic children; due to severe vitamin A deficiency.

---

enlargement

Word Building Example:

cephalomegaly
(cephalo-megaly)

Enlargement of the head.

-motor

General Terminology

-mimetic

General Terminology

Prefix
Combining Form
Suffix

-ole

Suffix

General Terminology

-oid

Suffix

General Terminology

Blood and the Immune System
Cardiovascular System
Endocrine System
Gastrointestinal System
General Terminology
Integumentary System

-one

Suffix

General Terminology

-oma (pl. -omata)

Suffix

General Terminology

Musculoskeletal System
Nervous System and Mental Health
Reproductive Systems
Respiratory System
The Senses
Urinary System

to move

Word Building Example:

algiomotor

(algio-motor)

Causing painful muscular contractions.

---

small, little, minute

Word Building Example:

bronchiole

(bronchi-ole)

One of approximately six generations of increasingly finer subdivisions of the bronchi, each smaller than 1 mm in diameter, and having no cartilage in its wall, but relatively abundant smooth muscle and elastic fibers.

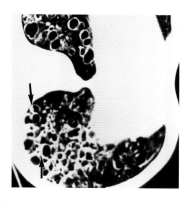

---

ketone group

---

mimicking, simulating

Word Building Example:

biomimetic

(bio-mimetic)

Imitative of biologic process or life.

---

resemblance to, equivalent to

---

tumor, neoplasm

Word Building Example:

hemorrhoid

(hemo-rrh-oid)

A varicose condition of the external hemorrhoidal veins causing painful swellings at the anus.

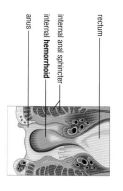

rectum

internal anal sphincter

internal **hemorrhoid**

anus

Word Building Example:

lactone

(lact-one)

An intramolecular organic anhydride formed from a hydroxyacid by the loss of water between a hydroxyl and a –COOH group.

Word Building Example:

myoma

(my-oma)

A benign neoplasm of muscular tissue.

-opia, -opsia

The Senses

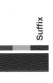

Suffix

-onium

General Terminology

Suffix

Prefix

Combining Form

Suffix

-orexia

Nervous System & Mental Health

Suffix

-opsy

General Terminology

Suffix

Blood and the Immune System

Cardiovascular System

Endocrine System

Gastrointestinal System

General Terminology

Integumentary System

-ose

General Terminology

Suffix

-ory

General Terminology

Suffix

Musculoskeletal System

Nervous System and Mental Health

Reproductive Systems

Respiratory System

The Senses

Urinary System

vision

myopia
(my-opia)

Word Building Example:

That optic condition in which parallel light rays are brought by the ocular media to focus in front of the retina.

positively charged radical

hydronium
(hydr-onium)

Word Building Example:

The hydrated proton, H_3O^+, a form in which hydrogen ion exists in aqueous solutions

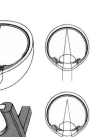
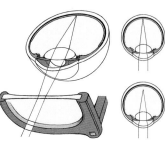

appetite

anorexia
(an-orexia)

Word Building Example:

Diminished appetite; aversion to food.

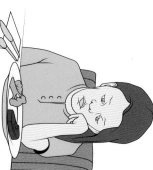
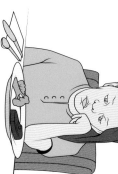

view

biopsy
(bi-opsy)

Word Building Example:

1. Process of removing tissue from living patients for macroscopic diagnostic examination. 2. A specimen obtained by brush or needle and syringe aspiration for biopsy.

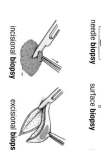

incisional **biopsy**

needle **biopsy**

surface **biopsy**

excisional **biopsy**

punch **biopsy**

full of, abounding

sucrose
(sucr-ose)

Word Building Example:

A nonreducing disaccharide made up of D-glucose and D-fructose obtained from sugar cane, *Saccharum officinarum*, from several species of sorghum, and from the sugar beet, *Beta vulgaris*.

pertaining to

sensory neuron
(sens-ory) neuron

Word Building Example:

A neuron conveying information originating from sensory receptors or nerve endings; an efferent neuron, may be a general or special sensory neuron.

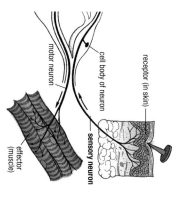

motor neuron

cell body of neuron

receptor (in skin)

sensory neuron

effector (muscle)

Card 211

-osis (pl. -oses)

General Terminology

Suffix

- Prefix
- Combining Form
- Suffix

Card 212

-osmia

The Senses

Suffix

Card 213

-ous

General Terminology

Suffix

- Blood and the Immune System
- Cardiovascular System
- Endocrine System
- Gastrointestinal System
- General Terminology
- Integumentary System

Card 214

-oxia

General Terminology

Suffix

Card 215

-para

Reproductive Systems

Suffix

- Musculoskeletal System
- Nervous System and Mental Health
- Reproductive Systems
- Respiratory System
- The Senses
- Urinary System

Card 216

-paresis

General Terminology

Suffix

sense of smell

Word Building Example:

euosmia
(eu-osmia)

1. A pleasant odor. 2. Normal olfaction.

oxygen

hypoxia
(hyp-oxia)

Lower than normal levels of oxygen in inspired gases, arterial blood, or tissue, short of anoxia.

Word Building Example:

partial or incomplete paralysis

hemiparesis
(hemi-paresis)

Weakness affecting one side of the body.

Word Building Example:

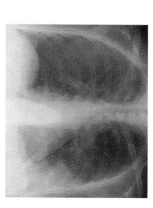

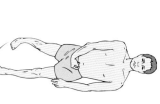
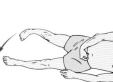

process, condition or state,
usually abnormal or diseased

scoliosis
(scoli-osis)

Abnormal lateral curvature of the vertebral column.

Word Building Example:

pertaining to

dizygous
(di-zyg-ous)

Relating to twins derived from two separate zygotes.

Word Building Example:

woman who has given birth

multipara
(multi-para)

A woman who has given birth at least twice to an infant, liveborn or not, weighing 500 g or more, or having an estimated length of gestation of at least 20 weeks.

Word Building Example:

Card 218

-parous

Reproductive Systems

Suffix

Card 217

-pareunia

Reproductive Systems

Prefix
Combining Form
Suffix

Suffix

Card 220

-pathy

General Terminology

Prefix

Suffix

Card 219

-partum

Reproductive Systems

General Terminology

Suffix

Blood and the Immune System
Cardiovascular System
Endocrine System
Gastrointestinal System
General Terminology
Integumentary System

Card 222

-pepsia

Gastrointestinal System

Suffix

Card 221

-penia

General Terminology

Suffix

Musculoskeletal System
Nervous System and Mental Health
Reproductive Systems
Respiratory System
The Senses
Urinary System

to bear, to bring forth

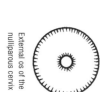

External os of the nulliparous cervix

coitus, sexual intercourse

---

nulliparous
(nulli-parous)

Having never borne children.

Word Building Example:

apareunia
(a-pareunia)

Absence or impossibility of coitus.

Word Building Example:

---

disease

birth

---

adenopathy
(adeno-pathy)

Swelling or morbid enlargement of the lymph nodes.

Word Building Example:

postpartum
(post-partum)

After childbirth.

Word Building Example:

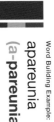

---

digestion

deficiency, decrease

---

dyspepsia
(dys-pepsia)

Impaired gastric function or "upset stomach" due to some stomach disorder.

Word Building Example:

pancytopenia
(pan-cyto-penia)

Pronounced reduction in the number of erythrocytes, leukocytes, and blood platelets in the circulating blood.

Word Building Example:

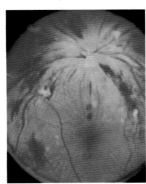

Card 223

-pexy

General Terminology

Suffix

Card 224

-phage, -phagia, -phagy

Gastrointestinal System

The Senses

Suffix

Card 225

-phasia

The Senses

Suffix

Card 226

-pheresis

General Terminology

Blood and the Immune System

Suffix

Card 227

-phil, -phile, -philia

Nervous System & Mental Health

Suffix

Card 228

-phobia

Nervous System & Mental Health

Suffix

eating, devouring

Word Building Example:

**lipophage
(lipo-phage)**

A cell that ingests fat.

the removal of

Word Building Example:

**plasmapheresis
(plasma-pheresis)**

Removal of whole blood from the body, separation of its cellular elements by centrifugation, and reinfusion of these elements in a suspension of saline or some other plasma substitute, thus depleting the body's own plasma without depleting its cells.

objectively unfounded morbid dread or fear

Word Building Example:

**ataxiophobia
(a-taxio-phobia)**

Morbid dread of disorder or untidiness.

fixation, usually surgical

Word Building Example:

**uteropexy
(utero-pexy)**

Fixation of a displaced or abnormally movable uterus.

speech

Word Building Example:

**dysphasia
(dys-phasia)**

Impairment in the production of speech and failure to arrange words clearly; caused by brain lesion.

affinity for, craving for, love

Word Building Example:

**hydrophil
(hydro-phil)**

A substance that attracts or associates with water molecules

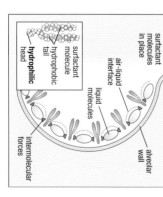

surfactant molecules in place

air–liquid interface

surfactant molecule

hydrophobic tail

hydrophilic head

liquid molecules

alveolar wall

intermolecular forces

-phoresis

General Terminology

Suffix

-phonia

The Senses

Prefix
Combining Form
Suffix

-phthisis

General Terminology

Suffix

-phrenia

General Terminology
Nervous System & Mental Health

Suffix

Blood and the Immune System
Cardiovascular System
Endocrine System
Gastrointestinal System
General Terminology
Integumentary System

-plakia

General Terminology

Suffix

-phylaxis

General Terminology

Suffix

Musculoskeletal System
Nervous System and Mental Health
Reproductive Systems
Respiratory System
The Senses
Urinary System

Word Building Example:

electrophoresis
(electro-phoresis)

The movement of particles in an electric field toward the anode or cathode.

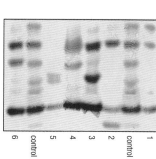

Word Building Example:

dysphonia
(dys-phonia)

Any disorder of phonation affecting voice quality or ability to produce voice.

---

wasting, atrophy

Word Building Example:

nephrophthisis
(nephro-phthisis)

Suppurative nephritis with wasting of the substance of the organ.

---

diaphragm;
the mind

Word Building Example:

schizophrenia
(schizo-phrenia)

A common type of psychosis characterized by abnormalities in perception, content of thought, and thought processes (hallucinations and delusions), and extensive withdrawal of one's interest from other people and the outside world, the investment of it being instead in one's own mental life.

---

plaque

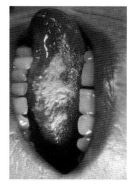

Word Building Example:

leukoplakia
(leuko-plakia)

A white patch of oral mucous membrane that cannot be wiped off and diagnosed clinically; the spots are smooth, irregular in size and shape, hard, and occasionally fissured.

---

protection against
infection

Word Building Example:

anaphylaxis
(ana-phylaxis)

The immediate, transient kind of allergic reaction characterized by contraction of smooth muscle and dilation of capillaries due to release of pharmacologically active substances (histamine, bradykinin, serotonin, and slow-reacting substance).

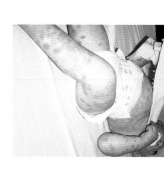

Card 236

-plasm

General Terminology

Suffix

Card 238

-plegia

Nervous System & Mental Health

Suffix

Card 240

-poiesis

Blood and the Immune System

Suffix

Card 235

-plasia

General Terminology

Suffix

Prefix

Combining Form

Suffix

Card 237

-plasty

General Terminology

Integumentary System

Suffix

Blood and the Immune System

Cardiovascular System

Endocrine System

Gastrointestinal System

General Terminology

Integumentary System

Card 239

-pnea

Respiratory System

Cardiovascular System

Suffix

Musculoskeletal System

Nervous System and Mental Health

Reproductive Systems

Respiratory System

The Senses

Urinary System

formation, growth substance

protoplasm
(proto-plasm)

1. Living matter, the substance of which animal and vegetable cells are formed. 2. The total cell material, including cell organelles.

paralysis

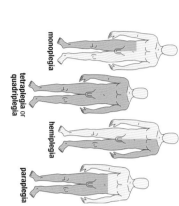

monoplegia

tetraplegia or quadriplegia

hemiplegia

paraplegia

Word Building Example:

paraplegia
(para-plegia)

Paralysis of both lower limbs and, generally, the lower trunk.

production, producing

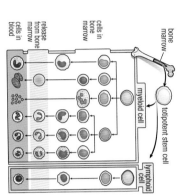

bone marrow

cells in bone marrow

release from bone marrow

cells in blood

myeloid cell

totipotent stem cell

lymphoid cell

Word Building Example:

hematopoiesis
(hemato-poiesis)

The process of formation and development of the various

---

formation (especially of cells)

Word Building Example:

dysplasia
(dys-plasia)

Abnormal tissue development.

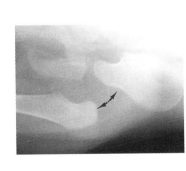

molding, shaping or the result thereof, as of a surgical procedure; surgical procedure for repair of a defect or restoration of form and/or function of a part

Word Building Example:

rhinoplasty
(rhino-plasty)

Reconstructive or cosmetic nasal surgery to correct form or function.

breath, respiration

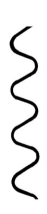

Word Building Example:

eupnea
(eu-pnea)

Easy, free respiration; the type observed in a normal individual under resting conditions.

-porosis

Musculoskeletal System

Suffix

-poietic

General Terminology

Prefix

Combining Form

Suffix

-praxia

Musculoskeletal System

Nervous System & Mental Health

Suffix

-prandial

Gastrointestinal System

Suffix

Blood and the Immune System

Cardiovascular System

Endocrine System

Gastrointestinal System

General Terminology

Integumentary System

-ptysis

Gastrointestinal System

Suffix

-ptosis

General Terminology

Suffix

Musculoskeletal System

Nervous System and Mental Health

Reproductive Systems

Respiratory System

The Senses

Urinary System

a porous condition

osteoporosis
(osteo-porosis)

Reduction in the quantity of bone or atrophy of skeletal tissue in postmenopausal women and older men.

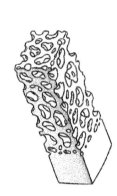

relating to formation

hematopoietic
(hemato-poietic)

Pertaining to or related to the formation of blood cells.

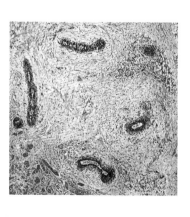

the performance
of an action

relating to a meal

apraxia
(a-praxia)

A disorder of voluntary movement, consisting of impairment in the performance of skilled or purposeful movements, notwithstanding the preservation of comprehension, muscular power, sensibility, and coordination in general.

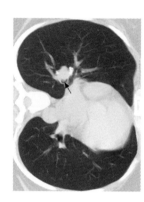

postprandial
(post-prandial)

Following a meal.

spitting

sinking down or
prolapse of an organ

hemoptysis
(hemo-ptysis)

The red respiratory protein of erythrocytes. SYN hemoglobin, hemoglobins.

gastroenteroptosis
(gastro-entero-ptosis)

Downward displacement of the stomach and a portion of the intestine.

-rrhaphy

General Terminology

Suffix

-rrhage, -rrhagia

General Terminology

Suffix

Prefix

Combining Form

Suffix

-rrhexis

General Terminology

Suffix

-rrhea

General Terminology

Suffix

Blood and the Immune System

Cardiovascular System

Endocrine System

Gastrointestinal System

General Terminology

Integumentary System

-schisis

General Terminology

Suffix

-salpinx

Reproductive Systems

Suffix

Musculoskeletal System

Nervous System and Mental Health

Reproductive Systems

Respiratory System

The Senses

Urinary System

surgical suturing

Word Building Example:
nephrorrhaphy
(nephro-rrhaphy)
Nephropexy by suturing the kidney.

excessive or unusual discharge, to burst forth

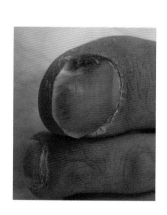

Word Building Example:
hemorrhage
(hemo-rrhage)
Blood convection or irrigation of tissues.

rupture

Word Building Example:
hepatorrhexis
(hepato-rrhexis)
Inflammation of the liver and biliary tree.

flowing, flux

Word Building Example:
diarrhea
(dia-rrhea)
An abnormally frequent discharge of semisolid or fluid fecal matter from the bowel.

fissure, splitting

Word Building Example:
plasmoschisis
(plasmo-schisis)
The splitting of protoplasm into fragments.

uterine tube, fallopian tube

Word Building Example:
hematosalpinx
(hemato-salpinx)
Collection of blood in a tube, often associated with a tubal pregnancy.

-scope

General Terminology

-sclerosis

General Terminology | Cardiovascular System

Suffix

Prefix

Combining Form

Suffix

-sect

General Terminology

Suffix

-scopy

General Terminology

Suffix

Blood and the Immune System

Cardiovascular System

Endocrine System

Gastrointestinal System

General Terminology

Integumentary System

-some

General Terminology

Suffix

-sis

General Terminology

Suffix

Musculoskeletal System

Nervous System and Mental Health

Reproductive Systems

Respiratory System

The Senses

Urinary System

instrument for viewing, but extended to include other methods of examination

Word Building Example:

endoscope
(endo-scope)

An instrument for the examination of the interior of a tubular or hollow organ.

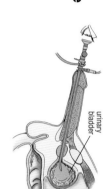

urinary bladder

to cut

Word Building Example:

bisect
(bi-sect)

To divide a body part into equal halves.

body, small body

Word Building Example:

chromosome
(chromo-some)

A body in the cell nucleus (of which there are normally 46 in humans) that is a bearer of genes.

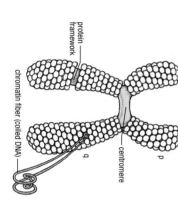

protein framework

chromatin fiber (coiled DNA)

centromere

p

q

hardening

Word Building Example:

tympanosclerosis
(tympano-sclerosis)

Formation of dense connective tissue in the middle ear, often causing hearing loss when the ossicles are involved.

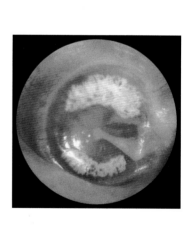

action or activity involving the use of an instrument for viewing

Word Building Example:

endoscopy
(endo-scopy)

Examination of the interior of a canal or hollow viscus by means of a special instrument, such as an endoscope.

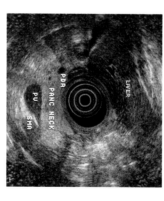

condition of

Word Building Example:

osmosis
(osmo-sis)

The process by which solvent tends to move through a semipermeable membrane from a solution of lower to a solution of higher osmolal concentration of the solutes to which the membrane is relatively impermeable.

high solute concentration, low fluid concentration and high osmotic pressure

low solute concentration, high fluid concentration and low osmotic pressure

FLUID

semipermeable membrane

-spasm

General Terminology

-spadias

Urinary System

Prefix

Combining Form

Suffix

-stasis

General Terminology

Suffix

-stalsis

General Terminology

Suffix

Blood and the Immune System

Cardiovascular System

Endocrine System

Gastrointestinal System

General Terminology

Integumentary System

-sthenia

General Terminology

Suffix

-static

General Terminology

Suffix

Musculoskeletal System

Nervous System and Mental Health

Reproductive Systems

Respiratory System

The Senses

Urinary System

sudden involuntary contraction of one or more muscles (includes cramps, contractures)

Word Building Example:

blepharospasm
(blepharo-spasm)

Involuntary spasmodic contraction of the orbicularis oculi muscle.

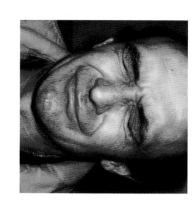

strength

Word Building Example:

hemostasis
(hemo-statis)

Denoting one of the tumors or varices constituting hemorrhoids.

stagnation of the blood or other fluids

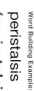

to tear or to gouge

phonasthenia
(phon-a-sthenia)

Word Building Example:

Difficult or abnormal voice production, the enunciation being too high, too loud, or too hard.

pyostatic
(pyo-static)

Word Building Example:

Arresting the formation of pus.

causing control

peristalsis
(peri-stalsis)

Word Building Example:

The movement of the intestine or other tubular structure, characterized by waves of alternate circular contraction and relaxation of the tube by which the contents are propelled onward.

contraction

hypospadias
(hypo-spadias)

Word Building Example:

A developmental anomaly characterized by a defect on the ventral surface of the penis so that the urethral opening is more proximal than normal.

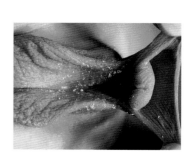

-tension

General Terminology

Suffix

-stomy

General Terminology
Gastrointestinal System

Prefix
Combining Form
Suffix

Suffix

-thorax

Musculoskeletal System
Respiratory System

Suffix

-therapy

General Terminology

Blood and the Immune System

Cardiovascular System

Endocrine System

Gastrointestinal System

General Terminology

Integumentary System

Suffix

-tic

General Terminology

Suffix

-thymia

Nervous System & Mental Health

Musculoskeletal System

Nervous System and Mental Health

Reproductive Systems

Respiratory System

The Senses

Urinary System

Suffix

to stretch, to tense

artificial or surgical opening

Word Building Example:

hypertension
(hyper-tension)

Persisting high arterial blood pressure; generally established guidelines are values exceeding 140 mmHg systolic or exceeding 90 mmHg diastolic blood pressure.

Word Building Example:

gastrojejunostomy
(gastro-jejuno-stomy)

Establishment of a direct communication between the stomach and the jejunum.

the upper part of the trunk between the neck and the abdomen

treatment of disease or disorder by any method

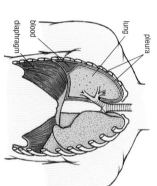

pleura

lung

blood

diaphragm

Word Building Example:

hemothorax
(hemo-thorax)

Arresting the flow of blood within the vessels.

Word Building Example:

chromotherapy
(chromo-therapy)

Treatment of disease by colored light.

pertaining to, relating to

mind, soul, emotions

Word Building Example:

aerobiotic
(aero-bio-tic)

Relating to an atmosphere containing oxygen.

Word Building Example:

dysthymia
(dys-thymia)

Chronic mood disorder manifested as depression for most of the day, more days than not, accompanied by some of the following symptoms: poor appetite or overeating, insomnia or hypersomnia, low energy or fatigue, low self-esteem, poor concentration, difficulty making decisions, and feelings of hopelessness.

-tocia

Reproductive Systems

Suffix

General Terminology

-tion, -ation

General Terminology

Suffix

Prefix

Combining Form

Suffix

-tomy

General Terminology

Suffix

General Terminology
Musculoskeletal System

-tome

General Terminology
Musculoskeletal System

Suffix

Blood and the Immune System

Cardiovascular System

Endocrine System

Gastrointestinal System

General Terminology

Integumentary System

-trichia

Integumentary System

Suffix

-tresia

General Terminology

Suffix

Musculoskeletal System

Nervous System and Mental Health

Reproductive Systems

Respiratory System

The Senses

Urinary System

childbirth

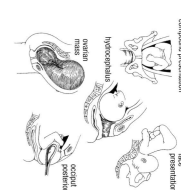

compound presentation

hydrocephalus

ovarian mass

face presentation

occiput posterior

process of

Word Building Example:

ovulation
(ovul-ation)

Release of an ovum from the ovarian follicle.

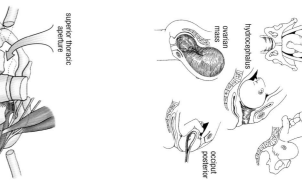

primary follicle

double-layered follicle

follicle at beginning of antrum formation

follicle approaching maturity

corpus albicans

corpus luteum

young corpus luteum

corpus hemorrhagicum

mature follicle

Word Building Example:

dystocia
(dys-tocia)

Difficult childbirth.

---

incision, a cutting operation

---

a cutting instrument

Word Building Example:

microtome
(micro-tome)

An instrument for making sections of biologic tissue for examination under the microscope.

---

condition or type of hair

Word Building Example:

thoracotomy
(thoraco-tomy)

Incision through the chest wall into the pleural space.

superior thoracic aperture

---

opening, hole

Word Building Example:

achromotrichia
(a-chromo-trichia)

Absence or loss of pigment in the hair.

Word Building Example:

atresia
(a-tresia)

Congenital absence of a normal opening or normally patent lumen.

-trite

General Terminology

Suffix

-tripsy

Urinary System

Suffix

Prefix

Combining Form

Suffix

-tropic

General Terminology

Suffix

-trophy

General Terminology

The Senses

Suffix

Blood and the Immune System

Cardiovascular System

Endocrine System

Gastrointestinal System

General Terminology

Integumentary System

-ula, -ule

General Terminology

Suffix

-type

General Terminology

Suffix

Musculoskeletal System

Nervous System and Mental Health

Reproductive Systems

Respiratory System

The Senses

Urinary System

to rub

Word Building Example:

lithotrite
(litho-trite)

A mechanical instrument used to crush a urinary calculus in lithotripsy.

---

a turning toward,
having an affinity for

Word Building Example:

hemotropic
(hemo-tropic)

Blood in the pleural cavity.

---

small, little

Word Building Example:

gastrula
(gastr-ula)

The embryo in the stage of development following the blastula or blastocyst formation.

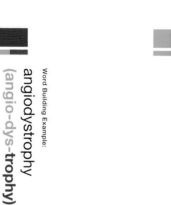

blastocele

archenteron

dorsal lip

yolk plug

Word Building Example:

hepaticolithotripsy
(hepatico-litho-tripsy)

Pertaining to the mechanism by which a substance in or on blood cells, especially the erythrocytes, attracts phagocytic cells.

---

food, nutrition

Word Building Example:

angiodystrophy
(angio-dys-trophy)

Defective formation or growth associated with marked vascular changes.

---

model

Word Building Example:

morphotype
(morpho-type)

An infra-subspecific group of bacterial strains distinguishable from other strains of the same species on the basis of morphologic characters that may or may not be associated with a change in serologic state.

-uretic

Urinary System

-um, -us

General Terminology

Prefix

Combining Form

Suffix

Suffix

-version

Reproductive Systems

The Senses

Suffix

-uria

Urinary System

Endocrine System

Suffix

Blood and the Immune System

Cardiovascular System

Endocrine System

Gastrointestinal System

General Terminology

Integumentary System

abdomin/o

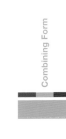

Combining Form

-y

Gastrointestinal System

Suffix

General Terminology

Suffix

Musculoskeletal System

Nervous System and Mental Health

Reproductive Systems

Respiratory System

The Senses

Urinary System

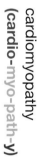

urine

Word Building Example:

diuretic

(di-uretic)

1. Promoting excretion of urine. 2. An agent that increases the amount of urine excreted.

turning

Word Building Example:

lateroversion

(latero-version)

Version to one side or the other, denoting especially a malposition of the uterus.

abdomen, abdominal

Word Building Example:

abdominoscopy

(abdomino-scopy)

Examination of the contents of the peritoneum with a peritoneoscope passed through the abdominal wall.

---

thing, singular noun ending

Word Building Example:

ileum

(ile-um)

The third portion of the small intestine, about 3.6 m (12 ft) in length, extending from the jejunum to the ileocecal opening.

urea; urine, urination

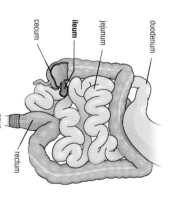

duodenum

jejunum

ileum

cecum

rectum

anus

Word Building Example:

dysuria

(dys-uria)

Difficulty or pain in urination.

condition of

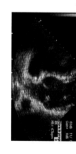

Word Building Example:

cardiomyopathy

(cardio-myo-path-y)

Disease of the myocardium; a primary disease of heart muscle in the absence of a known underlying etiology.

acanth/o

Musculoskeletal System

abort/i

Reproductive Systems

Prefix

Combining Form

Suffix

Combining Form

acous/o

Combining Form

The Senses

acetabul/o

Musculoskeletal System

Combining Form

Blood and the Immune System

Cardiovascular System

Endocrine System

Gastrointestinal System

General Terminology

Integumentary System

acromi/o

Combining Form

acr/o

General Terminology

Combining Form

Musculoskeletal System

Nervous System and Mental Health

Reproductive Systems

Respiratory System

The Senses

Urinary System

a spinous process; spiny, thorny

acanthoid
(acanth-oid)
Spine shaped.

Word Building Example:

hearing

acoustics
(acous-tics)
The science concerned with sounds and their perception.

Word Building Example:

acromion

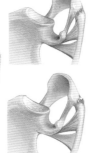
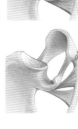

acromioclavicular separation
(acromio-clavicul-ar) separation
Injury to the ligaments that connect the clavicle to the shoulder bones (acromion).

Word Building Example:

abortion; miscarriage

abortigenic
(aborti-genic)
Producing abortion.

Word Building Example:

hip socket

acetabuloplasty
(acetabulo-plasty)
Any operation aimed at restoring the acetabulum to as near a normal state as possible.

Word Building Example:

extremity, end

acrodermatitis
(acro-dermat-itis)
Inflammation of the skin of the extremities.

Word Building Example:

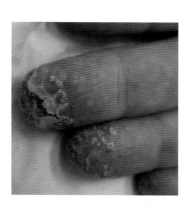

adenoid/o

Blood and the Immune System

Respiratory System

Combining Form

Endocrine System

aden/o

General Terminology

Endocrine System

Prefix

Combining Form

Suffix

Combining Form

adren/o, adrenal/o

Combining Form

General Terminology

Integumentary System

adip/o

Combining Form

Blood and the Immune System

Cardiovascular System

Endocrine System

Gastrointestinal System

General Terminology

Integumentary System

agglutin/o

Combining Form

General Terminology

aer/o

Combining Form

Musculoskeletal System

Nervous System and Mental Health

Reproductive Systems

Respiratory System

The Senses

Urinary System

adenoids

adenoidectomy
(adenoid-ectomy)

Surgery to remove adenoid tissue from the nasopharynx.

---

adrenal gland

---

adrenogenic
(adreno-genic)

Of adrenal origin.

---

adhere, form into
clumps

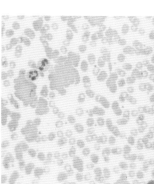

---

agglutination
(agglutin-ation)

The process by which suspended bacteria,
cells, or other particles are caused to adhere
and form clumps.

---

gland, glandular

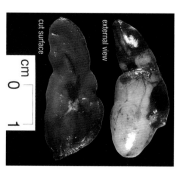

external view

cut surface

cm
0
1

---

adenoma
(aden-oma)

An ordinarily benign neoplasm of epithelial tissue in which the
tumor cells form glands or glandlike structures in the stroma.

---

fat, fatty

---

adipocyte
(adipo-cyte)

A connective tissue cell distended with one or
more fat globules.

---

air, gas

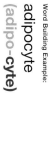

---

aerobic
(aero-bi-ic)

Living in air.

albin/o

General Terminology
Integumentary System

alg/o, algi/o,
algesi/o

General Terminology

Combining Form

alveol/o

Respiratory System

Combining Form

Combining Form

agor/a

Nervous System & Mental Health

Prefix

Combining Form

Suffix

Combining Form

albumin/o

Urinary System

Blood and the Immune System

Cardiovascular System

Endocrine System

Gastrointestinal System

General Terminology

Integumentary System

Combining Form

aliment/o

Gastrointestinal System

Musculoskeletal System

Nervous System and Mental Health

Reproductive Systems

Respiratory System

The Senses

Urinary System

Combining Form

white

Word Building Example:

albinism
(albin-ism)

Inherited (usually autosomal recessive) disorders with deficiency or absence of pigment in the skin, hair, and eyes, or eyes only, due to an abnormality in production of melanin.

pain

Word Building Example:

algesic
(alges-ic)

Painful; related to or causing pain.

the alveolar process;
concave vessel or bowl

Word Building Example:

alveolar abscess
(alveol-ar) abscess

An abscess situated within the alveolar process of the jaws, most often caused by extension of infection from an adjacent nonvital tooth.

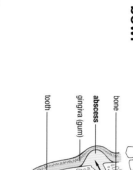

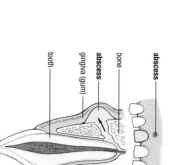

marketplace

Word Building Example:

agoraphobia
(agora-phobia)

A mental disorder characterized by an irrational fear of leaving a familiar setting.

protein

Word Building Example:

albuminuria
(albumin-uria)

Presence of protein in urine, chiefly albumin but also globulin.

nourish

Word Building Example:

alimentation
(aliment-ation)

Providing nourishment.

ambul/o

General Terminology

Combining Form

ambly/o

The Senses

Prefix

Combining Form

Suffix

---

amyl/o

Blood and the Immune System

Combining Form

amni/o

Reproductive Systems

Combining Form

Blood and the Immune System

Cardiovascular System

Endocrine System

Gastrointestinal System

General Terminology

Integumentary System

---

andr/o

Endocrine System

Combining Form

an/o

Gastrointestinal System

Combining Form

Musculoskeletal System

Nervous System and Mental Health

Reproductive Systems

Respiratory System

The Senses

Urinary System

to walk

Word Building Example:

ambulant

(ambul-ant)

Walking about or able to walk about.

---

starch

Word Building Example:

amyloidosis

(amyl-oid-osis)

A disease characterized by extracellular accumulation of amyloid in various organs and tissues of the body.

---

masculine, male

Word Building Example:

androgen

(andro-gen)

Generic term for an agent that stimulates activity of the accessory male sex organs, promotes development of male sex characteristics, or prevents changes in the latter that follow castration.

---

dullness, dimness, blunt

Word Building Example:

amblyopia

(ambly-opia)

Visual impairment not due to an ocular lesion and not fully correctable by an artificial lens.

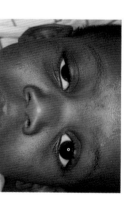

---

amnion (amniotic sac)

Word Building Example:

amnion

(amni-on)

Innermost of the extraembryonic membranes enveloping the embryo in utero and containing the amniotic fluid.

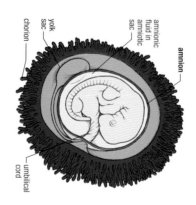

amnion

amniotic fluid in amniotic sac

yolk sac

chorion

umbilical cord

---

anus

Word Building Example:

anoplasty

(ano-plasty)

Plastic surgery of the anus.

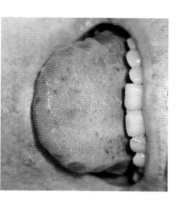

angi/o

Blood and the Immune System

Combining Form

aneurysm/o

Cardiovascular System

Prefix

Combining Form

Suffix

ankyl/o

Musculoskeletal System

Combining Form

anis/o

General Terminology

Combining Form

Blood and the Immune System

Cardiovascular System

Endocrine System

Gastrointestinal System

General Terminology

Integumentary System

anthrac/o

General Terminology

Combining Form

anter/o

General Terminology

Combining Form

Musculoskeletal System

Nervous System and Mental Health

Reproductive Systems

Respiratory System

The Senses

Urinary System

blood or lymph
vessels

angiography
(angio-graphy)

Radiography of vessels after the injection of a radiopaque
contrast material; usually requires percutaneous
insertion of a radiopaque catheter and positioning under
fluoroscopic control.

bent, crooked, stiff, fused,
fixed, closed

coal, carbon

ankylosis
(ankyl-osis)

Stiffening or fixation of a joint as the result of a
disease process, with fibrous or bony union
across the joint.

anthracosilicosis
(anthraco-silic-osis)

Pneumonoconiosis from accumulation of carbon and
silica in the lungs from inhaled coal dust.

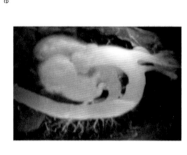

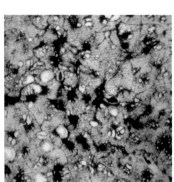

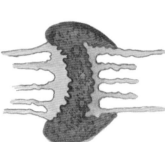

aneurysm

aneurysmotomy
(aneurysmo-tomy)

Incision into the sac of an aneurysm.

unequal, dissimilar, unlike

anisochromatic
(aniso-chroma-tic)

Not uniformly of one color.

anterior, front

anteroposterior
(antero-posteri-or)

Relating to both front and rear. In X-ray imaging,
describing the direction of the beam through the
patient from anterior to posterior.

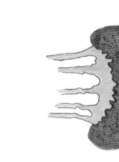

anteroposterior (AP)

Nervous System & Mental Health

Combining Form

anxi/o

General Terminology

Prefix

Combining Form

Suffix

anthrop/o

Gastrointestinal System

Combining Form

append/o,
appendic/o

Cardiovascular System

Combining Form

aort/o

Blood and the Immune System

Cardiovascular System

Endocrine System

Gastrointestinal System

General Terminology

Integumentary System

General Terminology

Combining Form

arch/e, archi/o

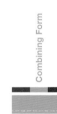

The Senses

Combining Form

aque/o

Musculoskeletal System

Nervous System and Mental Health

Reproductive Systems

Respiratory System

The Senses

Urinary System

uneasy, distressed, anxious

anxiolytic
(anxio-lytic)

Word Building Example:

Something that diminishes anxiety (e.g., a drug).

appendix

appendectomy
(append-ectomy)

Word Building Example:

Surgical removal of the vermiform appendix.

first, chief, extreme; primitive, ancestral

archeokinetic
(archeo-kine-tic)

Word Building Example:

Denoting a low and primordial type of motor nerve mechanism, such as is found in the peripheral and the ganglionic nervous systems.

involving human beings

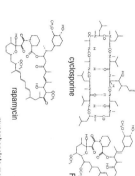

rapamycin

cyclosporine

mycophenolate mofetil (mycophenolic acid morpholinoethyl ester, RS-61443)

FK506

anthropocentric
(anthropo-centr-ic)

Word Building Example:

With a human bias, under the assumption that humankind is the central fact of the universe.

aorta

aortoplasty
(aorto-plasty)

Word Building Example:

A procedure for surgical repair of the aorta.

water

aqueduct
(aque-duct)

Word Building Example:

A conduit or canal.

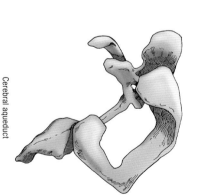

Cerebral aqueduct

arteriol/o

Cardiovascular System

arter/o, arteri/o

Cardiovascular System

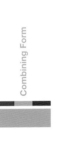

Prefix

Combining Form

Suffix

articul/o

Combining Form

Musculoskeletal System

arthr/o

Combining Form

Musculoskeletal System

Blood and the Immune System

Cardiovascular System

Endocrine System

Gastrointestinal System

General Terminology

Integumentary System

astr/o

Combining Form

General Terminolgy

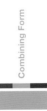

asbest/o

Combining Form

Respiratory System

Musculoskeletal System

Nervous System and Mental Health

Reproductive Systems

Respiratory System

The Senses

Urinary System

arteriole

Word Building Example:

arteriogram
(arterio-gram)

Radiographic demonstration of an artery after injection of contrast medium into it.

---

joint

Word Building Example:

articular capsule
(articul-ar) capsule

A sac enclosing the articulating ends of the bones participating in a synovial joint, formed by an outer fibrous articular capsule and an inner synovial membrane.

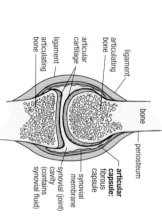

---

star

astrocyte
(astro-cyte)

Word Building Example:

One of the large neuroglia cells of nervous tissue.

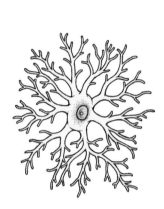

---

artery

Word Building Example:

arteriosclerosis
(arterio-scler-osis)

Hardening of the arteries.

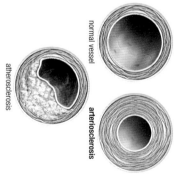

---

a joint, an articulation

arthroplasty
(arthro-plasty)

Word Building Example:

1. Creation of an artificial joint to correct ankylosis.
2. An operation to restore as far as possible the integrity and functional power of a joint.

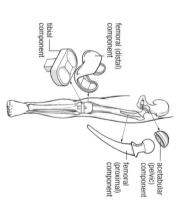

---

asbestos

asbestosis
(asbest-osis)

Word Building Example:

Pneumoconiosis due to inhalation of asbestos fibers suspended in the ambient air.

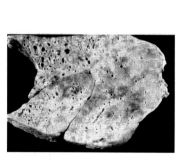

ather/o

Cardiovascular System

atel/o

Respiratory System

Prefix

Combining Form

Suffix

atri/o

Combining Form

Cardiovascular System

atlant/o, atl/o

Combining Form

General Terminology

Blood and the Immune System

Cardiovascular System

Endocrine System

Gastrointestinal System

General Terminology

Integumentary System

aur/i, aur/o, auricul/o

Combining Form

The Senses

audi/o, audit/o

Combining Form

The Senses

Musculoskeletal System

Nervous System and Mental Health

Reproductive Systems

Respiratory System

The Senses

Urinary System

soft, pasty

Word Building Example:
atherectomy
(ather-ectomy)

Invasive removal of an atheroma or plaque from an artery.

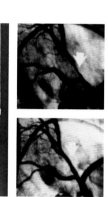

incomplete

Word Building Example:
atelectasis
(atel-ectasis)

Reduction or absence of air in part or all of a lung, with resulting loss of lung volume.

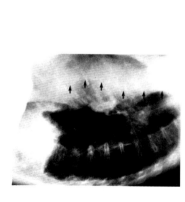

the atrium, atrial

Word Building Example:
atriomegaly
(atrio-megaly)

Enlargement of the atrium.

atlas

Word Building Example:
atlantoaxial
(atlanto-axi-al)

Pertaining to the atlas and the axis; denoting the joint between the first two cervical vertebrae.

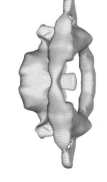

ear

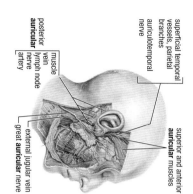

superficial temporal vessels, parietal branches

auriculotemporal nerve

posterior **auricular** muscle vein lymph node nerve artery

external jugular vein great **auricular** nerve

superior and anterior **auricular** muscles

sense of hearing

Word Building Example:
audiogram
(audio-gram)

The graphic record drawn from the results of hearing tests with the audiometer.

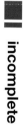

hearing-threshold level in decibels

frequency in cycles per second (Hertz)

key: right ◯ left ✕

auricular
(auricul-ar)

Relating to the ear, or to an auricle in any sense.

axill/o

General Terminology

Combining Form

ax/o

General Terminology

- Prefix
- Combining Form
- Suffix

---

bacill/i, bacill/o

General Terminology

Combining Form

az/o, azot/o

Combining Form

General Terminology

- Blood and the Immune System
- Cardiovascular System
- Endocrine System
- Gastrointestinal System
- General Terminology
- Integumentary System

---

balan/o

Combining Form

Urinary System
Endocrine System

Combining Form

bacteri/o

General Terminology

Combining Form

- Musculoskeletal System
- Nervous System and Mental Health
- Reproductive Systems
- Respiratory System
- The Senses
- Urinary System

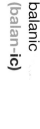

armpit

axis

Word Building Example:

axillary artery
(axill-ary) artery

The continuation of the subclavian artery after it crosses the first rib to enter the axilla; it becomes the brachial artery on passing the interior border of the teres major muscle.

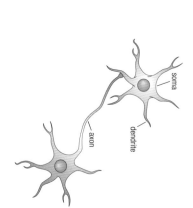

supreme thoracic artery
thoracoacromial trunk
circumflex humeral arteries
lateral thoracic artery
subscapular artery

bacillus

Word Building Example:

axodendritic
(axo-dendri-tic)

Pertaining to the synaptic relationship of an axon with a dendrite of another neuron.

soma
dendrite
axon

nitrogenous compound

---

bacilliform
(bacilli-form)

Rod-shaped.

Word Building Example:

azoturia
(azot-uria)

An increased elimination of urea in the urine.

glans penis

Word Building Example:

bacteriophage
(bacterio-phage)

A virus with specific affinity for bacteria, found in association with nearly all groups of bacteria.

bacterial cell membrane
viral DNA
bacterial cytoplasm
tail fibers
core
tail sheath
protein coat
viral DNA

bacterium

Word Building Example:

balanic
(balan-ic)

Relating to the glans penis or glans clitoridis.

bar/o

General Terminology

Prefix

Combining Form

Suffix

bas/o

Blood and the Immune System

Combining Form

bil/i

Gastrointestinal System

Blood and the Immune System

Cardiovascular System

Endocrine System

Gastrointestinal System

General Terminology

Integumentary System

bilirubin/o

Gastrointestinal System

Combining Form

blast/o

General Terminology

Musculoskeletal System

Nervous System and Mental Health

Reproductive Systems

Respiratory System

The Senses

Urinary System

blenn/o

Respiratory System

Combining Form

base;
basis

Word Building Example:

basophil

(baso-phil)

A cell with granules that stain specifically with basic dyes.

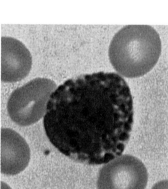

---

yellow bile pigment, bilirubin

Word Building Example:

bilirubinemia

(bilirubin-emia)

The presence of increased amounts of bilirubin in the blood, where it is normally present in only relatively small amounts.

---

mucus

---

pressure

Word Building Example:

baroreceptor

(baro-recept-or)

1. In general, any sensor of pressure changes.
2. Sensory nerve endings in the wall of the atrium of the heart, vena cava, aortic arch, and carotid sinus, sensitive to stretching of the wall resulting from increased pressure from within and functioning as the receptor of central reflex mechanisms that tend to reduce that pressure.

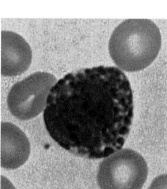

vagus nerve
carotid body
carotid sinus
common carotid
artery
brachiocephalic
artery
aortic arch
baroreceptors
baroreceptors
glossopharyngeal nerve

---

bile

Word Building Example:

biligenesis

(bile-genesis)

Bile production.

---

process of budding
by cells or tissue

Word Building Example:

blastocyst

(blasto-cyst)

The modified blastula stage of mammalian embryos (including human), consisting of the embryoblast (inner cell mass) and a thin trophoblast layer enclosing the blastocystic cavity.

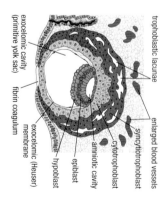

trophoblastic lacunae
exocoelomic cavity
(primitive yolk sac)
fibrin coagulum
exocoelomic (Heuser)
membrane
hypoblast
epiblast
amniotic cavity
cytotrophoblast
syncytiotrophoblast
enlarged blood vessels

Word Building Example:

blennoid

(blenn-oid)

Resembling mucus.

bol/o

General Terminology

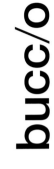

blephar/o

The Senses

Prefix

Combining Form

Suffix

bronch/i, bronch/o

Combining Form

Respiratory System

brachi/o

Combining Form

Musculoskeletal System

Cardiovascular System

Blood and the Immune System

Cardiovascular System

Endocrine System

Gastrointestinal System

General Terminology

Integumentary System

bucc/o

Combining Form

Gastrointestinal System

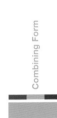

bronchiol/o

Combining Form

Respiratory System

Musculoskeletal System

Nervous System and Mental Health

Reproductive Systems

Respiratory System

The Senses

Urinary System

throw, cast

Word Building Example:
bolometer
(bolo-meter)

An instrument for determining minute degrees of radiant heat.

bronchus

Word Building Example:
bronchocele
(broncho-cele)

A circumscribed dilation of a bronchus.

cheek

Word Building Example:
buccolabial
(bucco-labi-al)

Relating to both cheek and lip dentistry referring to that aspect of the dental arch or those surfaces of the teeth in contact with the mucosa of lip and cheek.

eyelid

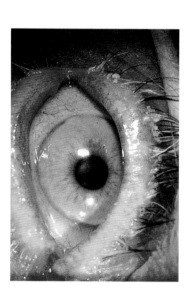

Word Building Example:
blepharitis
(blephar-itis)

Inflammation of the eyelids.

arm

Word Building Example:
brachiocephalic vein
(brachio-cephal-ic) vein

Two veins on either side of the neck formed by the junction of the internal jugular and subclavian veins. They drain from the head, neck, and upper extremities and unite to form the superior vena cava.

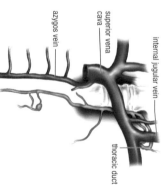

internal jugular vein

superior vena cava

azygos vein

thoracic duct

bronchiole

Word Building Example:
bronchiolitis
(bronchiol-itis)

Inflammation of the bronchioles, often associated with bronchopneumonia.

byssin/o

Respiratory System

calcane/o

Combining Form

Musculoskeletal System

capn/o, carb/o

Combining Form

burs/o

Musculoskeletal System

Prefix

Combining Form

Suffix

calc/i

Combining Form

General Terminology

Musculoskeletal System

Blood and the Immune System

Cardiovascular System

Endocrine System

Gastrointestinal System

General Terminology

Integumentary System

cali/o, calic/o

Combining Form

Urinary System

Musculoskeletal System

Nervous System and Mental Health

Reproductive Systems

Respiratory System

The Senses

Urinary System

cotton dust

bursa, fluid-containing closed sac or envelope

---

byssinosis
(byssin-osis)

Obstructive airway disease in people who work with unprocessed cotton, flax, or hemp; caused by reaction to material in the dust.

Word Building Example:

---

bursopathy
(burso-pathy)

Any disease of a bursa.

Word Building Example:

---

calcaneus, heel

---

calcium

---

calcaneodynia
(calcaneo-dynia)

A condition in which bearing weight on the heel causes pain of varying severity.

Word Building Example:

---

calcification
(calci-fication)

1. Deposition of lime or other insoluble calcium salts. 2. A process in which tissue or noncellular material in the body becomes hardened as the result of precipitates or larger deposits of insoluble salts of calcium (and also magnesium), especially calcium carbonate and phosphate (hydroxyapatite) normally occurring only in the formation of bone and teeth.

Word Building Example:

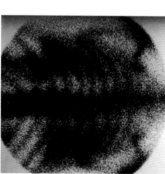

---

carbon dioxide

---

calix

---

capnograph
(capno-graph)

Instrument by which a continuous graph of the carbon dioxide content of expired air is obtained.

Word Building Example:

---

calicotomy
(calico-tomy)

Incision into a calyx, usually for removal of a calculus.

Word Building Example:

cardi/o

Cardiovascular System
Gastrointestinal System

carcin/o

General Terminology

Combining Form

Prefix
Combining Form
Suffix

caud/o

Combining Form

General Terminology

carp/i, carp/o

Combining Form

Musculoskeletal System

Blood and the Immune System
Cardiovascular System
Endocrine System
Gastrointestinal System
General Terminology
Integumentary System

cauter/o

Combining Form

caus/o

Combining Form

General Terminology

Musculoskeletal System
Nervous System and Mental Health
Reproductive Systems
Respiratory System
The Senses
Urinary System

heart; esophageal opening of stomach

cardiopulmonary
(cardio-pulmon-ary)

Relating to the heart and lungs. SYN: pneumocardial.

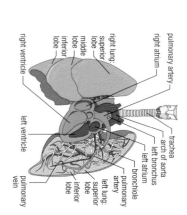

right lung:
superior lobe
middle lobe
inferior lobe

pulmonary artery
right atrium

trachea
arch of aorta
left bronchus
left atrium
bronchiole
pulmonary artery
left lung:
superior lobe
inferior lobe
pulmonary vein

left ventricle
right ventricle

---

cancer

Word Building Example:

carcinoma
(carcin-oma)

Any of the various types of malignant neoplasm derived from epithelial tissue, occurring more frequently in the skin and large intestine in both sexes, the lung and prostate gland in men, and the lung and breast in women.

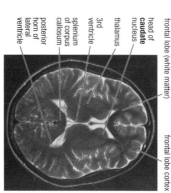

---

tail, lower part of body

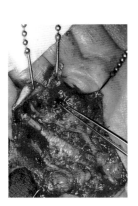

frontal lobe (white matter)

posterior horn of lateral ventricle
splenium of corpus callosum
3rd ventricle
thalamus
head of **caudate** nucleus

frontal lobe cortex

Word Building Example:

caudate
(caud-ate)

Tailed; possessing a tail.

---

wrist bone

Word Building Example:

carpectomy
(carp-ectomy)

Partial or total carpal excision.

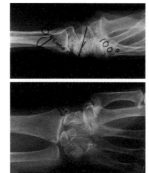

---

to burn

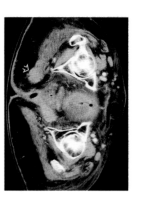

Word Building Example:

cauterization
(cauter-ization)

The act of scarring, burning, or cutting the skin or other tissues by means of heat, cold, electric current, ultrasound, or caustic chemicals.

---

burn, burning, hot

Word Building Example:

caustic
(caus-tic)

1. Exerting an effect resembling a burn. 2. An agent producing this effect. 3. Denoting a solution of a strong alkali (e.g., caustic soda).

Card 368

celi/o

Gastrointestinal System

Combining Form

Card 367

cec/o

Gastrointestinal System

Prefix

Combining Form

Suffix

Card 370

cephal/o

Combining Form

General Terminology

Card 369

centr/i

Combining Form

General Terminology

Blood and the Immune System

Cardiovascular System

Endocrine System

Gastrointestinal System

General Terminology

Integumentary System

Card 372

cerebr/i, cerebr/o

Nervous System & Mental Health

Combining Form

Card 371

cerebell/o

Combining Form

Nervous System & Mental Health

Cardiovascular System

Musculoskeletal System

Nervous System and Mental Health

Reproductive Systems

Respiratory System

The Senses

Urinary System

abdomen

---

cecum

Word Building Example:

celiotomy
(celio-tomy)

Transabdominal incision into the peritoneal cavity.

Word Building Example:

cecitis
(cec-itis)

Inflammation of the cecum.

---

head, toward the head

---

center

Word Building Example:

cephalhematoma
(cephal-hemat-oma)

An effusion of blood beneath the periosteum of a cranial bone, seen frequently in a newborn as a result of birth trauma.

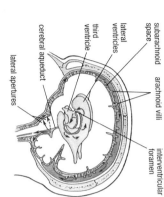

Word Building Example:

centriole
(centri-ole)

Tubular structures, 150 nm by 300–500 nm, with a wall having nine triple microtubules, usually seen as paired organelles lying in the cytocentrum.

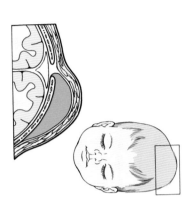

---

cerebrum, brain

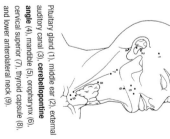

subarachnoid space

arachnoid villi

lateral ventricles

third ventricle

interventricular foramen

cerebral aqueduct

lateral apertures

---

cerebellum

Word Building Example:

cerebrospinal fluid
(cerebro-spin-al) fluid

A fluid largely secreted by the choroid plexuses of the ventricles of the brain, filling the ventricles and the subarachnoid cavities of the brain and spinal cord.

Word Building Example:

cerebellopontine angle
(cerebello-pont-ine) angle

The angle formed at the junction of the cerebellum, pons, and medulla.

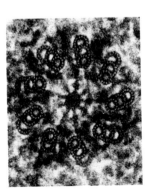

Pituitary gland (1), middle ear (2), external auditory canal (3), mandible (5), oropharynx (6), cervical superior (7), thyroid capsule (8), and lower anterolateral neck (9). **cerebellopontine angle** (4),

cheil/o

The Senses

cervic/o

Musculoskeletal System

Reproductive Systems

Prefix

Combining Form

Suffix

chir/o

Combining Form

Musculoskeletal System

chem/o

Combining Form

General Terminology

Blood and the Immune System

Cardiovascular System

Endocrine System

Gastrointestinal System

General Terminology

Integumentary System

chol/e, chol/o

Combining Form

Combining Form

Gastrointestinal System

chlor/o

Combining Form

General Terminology

Musculoskeletal System

Nervous System and Mental Health

Reproductive Systems

Respiratory System

The Senses

Urinary System

lips

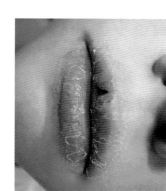

Word Building Example:

cheilitis
(cheil-itis)

Inflammation of the lips or lip.

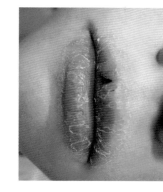

hand

Word Building Example:

chiromegaly
(chiro-megaly)

A condition characterized by abnormally large hands.

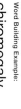

bile

Word Building Example:

cholemesis
(chol-emesis)

Vomiting of bile.

---

a cervix or neck, in any sense

Word Building Example:

cervicitis
(cervic-itis)

Inflammation of the mucous membrane, frequently involving also the deeper structures, of the cervix uteri.

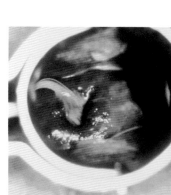

chemistry

Word Building Example:

chemotherapy
(chemo-therapy)

Treatment of disease by means of chemical substances or drugs; usually used in reference to neoplastic disease.

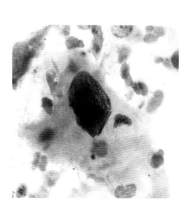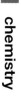

green

Word Building Example:

hyperchlorhydria
(hyper-chlor-hydr-ia)

Presence of an excessive amount of hydrochloric acid in the stomach.

Card
380

Card
379

Card
382

Card
381

Card
384

Card
383

cholecyst/o

Gastrointestinal System

Combining Form

chondr/o, chondri/o

Musculoskeletal System

Combining Form

chrom/o, chromat/o

General Terminology

Combining Form

cholangi/o

Gastrointestinal System

Combining Form

Prefix

Combining Form

Suffix

choledoch/o

Gastrointestinal System

Combining Form

Blood and the Immune System

Cardiovascular System

Endocrine System

Gastrointestinal System

General Terminology

Integumentary System

chori/o, choroid/o

General Terminology

Reproductive Systems

Combining Form

Musculoskeletal System

Nervous System and Mental Health

Reproductive Systems

Respiratory System

The Senses

Urinary System

Word Building Example:

cholecystectomy
(chole-cyst-ectomy)

Surgical removal of the gallbladder.

---

cartilage

Word Building Example:

chondrodynia
(chondro-dynia)

Pain in cartilage.

---

color

Word Building Example:

chromatophore
(chromato-phore)

1. A plastid, colored because of the presence of chlorophyll or other pigments, found in certain forms of protozoa.
2. Melanophage: a pigment-bearing phagocyte found chiefly in the skin, mucous membrane, and choroid coat of the eye, and also in melanomas.

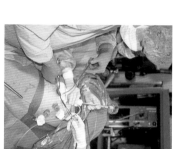

Word Building Example:

colonography
(colono-graphy)

Imaging study of the colon, most often using CT or MRI.

---

common bile duct

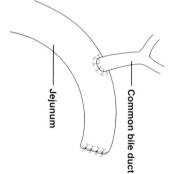

Jejunum

Common bile duct

Word Building Example:

choledochojejunostomy
(choledocho-jejuno-stomy)

Anastomosis between the common bile duct and the jejunum.

---

any membrane,
especially that which
encloses the fetus

Word Building Example:

choroid
(chor-oid)

The middle vascular tunic of the eye lying between the retina and the sclera.

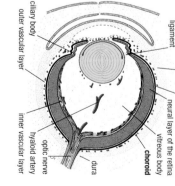

ciliary body
outer vascular layer

suspensory ligament

sclera
pigment layer of the retina
neural layer of the retina
vitreous body
choroid

optic nerve
hyaloid artery
inner vascular layer

dura

chron/o

General Terminology

Prefix

Combining Form

Suffix

Combining Form

chyl/o, chyl/i

Gastrointestinal System

cirrh/o

Gastrointestinal System

Blood and the Immune System

Cardiovascular System

Endocrine System

Gastrointestinal System

General Terminology

Integumentary System

Combining Form

cis/o

General Terminology

Combining Form

Combining Form

claustr/o

General Terminology

Musculoskeletal System

Nervous System and Mental Health

Reproductive Systems

Respiratory System

The Senses

Urinary System

Combining Form

clavicul/o

Musculoskeletal System

Combining Form

juice

chylothorax
(chylo-thorax)

An accumulation of milky chylous fluid in the pleural space, usually on the left.

---

to cut

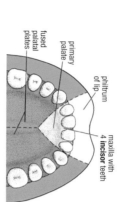

fused palatal plates
primary palate
philtrum of lip
maxilla with **4 incisor** teeth

incisor
(in-cis-or)

A tooth with a chisel-shaped crown and a single conical tapering root; there are four of these teeth in the anterior part of each jaw, in both the deciduous and the permanent dentitions.

---

clavicle

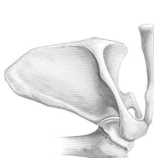

clavicular notch of sternum
(clavicul-ar) notch of sternum

A hollow on either side of the upper surface of the manubrium sterni that articulates with the clavicle.

---

time

chronobiology
(chrono-bio-logy)

That aspect of biology concerned with the timing of biologic events, especially repetitive or cyclic phenomena.

---

orange/yellow

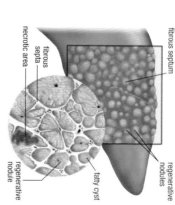

fibrous septum
fibrous septa
necrotic area
regenerative nodule
fatty cyst
regenerative nodules

cirrhosis
(cirrho-sis)

Liver disease characterized by diffuse damage to hepatic parenchymal cells, with nodular regeneration, fibrosis, and disturbance of normal architecture; associated with failure in the function of hepatic cells and interference with blood flow in the liver, frequently resulting in jaundice, portal hypertension, ascites, and ultimately biochemical and functional signs of hepatic failure.

---

enclosed space

claustrophobia
(claustro-phobia)

A morbid fear of being in a confined place.

clon/o

General Terminology

Combining Form

clitor/o,
clitorid/o

Urinary System

Prefix

Combining Form

Suffix

coccy, coccyg/o

Musculoskeletal System

Combining Form

coagul/o

Blood and the Immune System

Combining Form

Blood and the Immune System

Cardiovascular System

Endocrine System

Gastrointestinal System

General Terminology

Integumentary System

col/o, colon/o

Gastrointestinal System

Combining Form

cochle/o

The Senses

Combining Form

Musculoskeletal System

Nervous System and Mental Health

Reproductive Systems

Respiratory System

The Senses

Urinary System

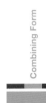

clitoris

Word Building Example:

clitorism
(clitor-ism)

Prolonged and usually painful erection of the clitoris; the female analogue of priapism.

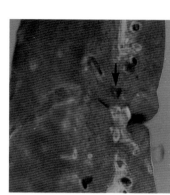

clotting

clone

Word Building Example:

clonorchiasis
(clon-orch-iasis)

A disease caused by the fluke *Clonorchis sinensis*, affecting the distal bile ducts after ingestion of raw, smoked, or undercooked fish or raw crayfish.

coccyx

Word Building Example:

coccygodynia
(coccygo-dynia)

Pain in the coccygeal region.

colon

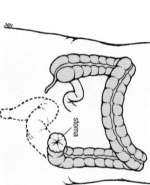

stoma

Word Building Example:

colostomy
(colo-stomy)

Establishment surgically of an artificial cutaneous opening into the colon.

Word Building Example:

coagulant
(coagul-ant)

An agent that causes, stimulates, or accelerates coagulation, especially with reference to blood.

cochlea (of inner ear)

Word Building Example:

cochlear implant
(cochle-ar) implant

Auditory amplification device surgically implanted with its stimulating electrodes inserted directly into the nonfunctioning cochlea.

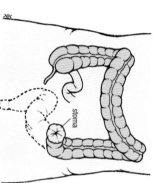

external coil
internal coil
ground electrode in epitympanum
microphone
stimulator wire from microphone
stimulator wire from speech processor to external coil
pharyngotympanic tube
ear drum
cochlear nerve
cochlea
active electrode

condyl/o

Musculoskeletal System

colp/o

Reproductive Systems

Urinary System

Prefix

Combining Form

Suffix

conjunctiv/o

Combining Form

The Senses

coni/o

Combining Form

General Terminology

Blood and the Immune System

Cardiovascular System

Endocrine System

Gastrointestinal System

General Terminology

Integumentary System

corne/o

Combining Form

cor/o, core/o

Combining Form

The Senses

Musculoskeletal System

Nervous System and Mental Health

Reproductive Systems

Respiratory System

The Senses

Urinary System

rounded articular surface at the extremity of a bone

vagina

Word Building Example:
**condylotomy
(condylo-tomy)**

Division, without removal, of a condyle.

Word Building Example:
**colporectopexy
(colpo-recto-pexy)**

Repair of a prolapsed rectum by suturing it to the wall of the vagina.

conjunctiva

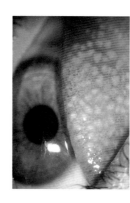

dust

Word Building Example:
**conjunctivitis
(conjunctiv-itis)**

Disorder in which the conjunctivae are reddened. The eyes tear and produce exudate along the eyelid; may progress to drooping of the eyelid such that abnormal tissue may form.

Word Building Example:
**coniofibrosis
(conio-fibr-osis)**

Fibrosis produced by dust, especially of the lungs by inhaled dust.

cornea

pupil

Word Building Example:
**corneosclera
(corneo-sclera)**

Combined cornea and sclera considered as forming the eyeball's external coat.

Word Building Example:
**corelysis
(core-lysis)**

A rarely used term for freeing of adhesions between lens capsule and the iris.

coron/o

Cardiovascular System

Combining Form

Prefix

Combining Form

Suffix

cortic/o

Endocrine System

cost/o

Musculoskeletal System

Combining Form

Blood and the Immune System

Cardiovascular System

Endocrine System

Gastrointestinal System

General Terminology

Integumentary System

crani/o

Nervous System & Mental Health

Musculoskeletal System

Combining Form

crin/o

Endocrine System

Combining Form

Musculoskeletal System

Nervous System and Mental Health

Reproductive Systems

Respiratory System

The Senses

Urinary System

cruci/o

General Terminology

Combining Form

cortex

Word Building Example:

cortilymph
(corti-lymph)

The fluid in the Corti tunnel.

circle or crown

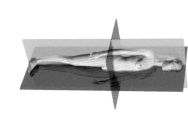

coronal

Word Building Example:

coronal
(coron-al)

Relating to a corona or the coronal plane.

cranium, skull

ribs

cross-shaped

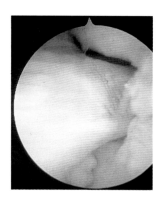

to secrete

Word Building Example:

cranioschisis
(cranio-schisis)

Congenital malformation with incomplete closure of the cranium; often accompanied by grossly defective development of the brain.

Word Building Example:

costectomy
(cost-ectomy)

Excision of a rib.

Word Building Example:

cruciate ligament
(cruci-ate) ligament

Ligament shaped like, or resembling, a cross.

Word Building Example:

endocrinoma
(endo-crin-oma)

A tumor with endocrine tissue that retains the function of the parent organ, usually to an excessive degree.

Card
409

crypt/o

Card
410

General Terminology
Urinary System

Combining Form

cry/o

General Terminology

Prefix

Combining Form

Suffix

Combining Form

Card
411

cutane/o

Card
412

General Terminology
Integumentary System

Combining Form

culd/o

Reproductive Systems

Blood and the Immune System

Cardiovascular System

Endocrine System

Gastrointestinal System

General Terminology

Integumentary System

Combining Form

Card
413

cycl/o

Card
414

The Senses

Combining Form

cyan/o

General Terminology

Musculoskeletal System

Nervous System and Mental Health

Reproductive Systems

Respiratory System

The Senses

Urinary System

Combining Form

hidden

cryptogenic
(crypto-genic)

Of obscure, indeterminate etiology or origin, in contrast to phanerogenic.

---

cold

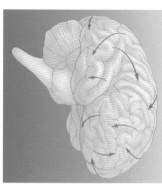

cryoanesthesia
(cryo-ana-esthesia)

Localized application of cold as a means of producing regional anesthesia.

---

skin

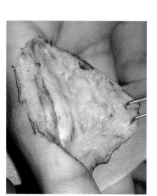

subcutaneous
(sub-cutane-ous)

Beneath the skin.

---

circle, cycle;
ciliary body

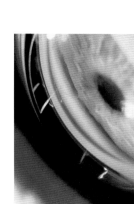

cyclodialysis
(cyclo-dia-lysis)

Establishment of a communication between the anterior chamber and the suprachoroidal space to reduce intraocular pressure in glaucoma.

---

cul-de-sac

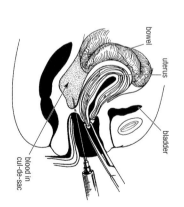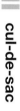

bowel

uterus

bladder

blood in
cul-de-sac

culdocentesis
(culdo-centesis)

Aspiration of fluid from the cul-de-sac by puncture of the vaginal vault near the midline between the uterosacral ligaments.

---

blue

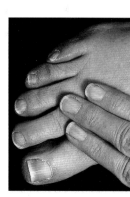

cyanosis
(cyan-osis)

A dark bluish or purplish discoloration of the skin and mucous membrane due to deficient oxygenation of the blood, evident when reduced hemoglobin in the blood exceeds 5 g/100 mL.

dacry/o

The Senses

General Terminology

Combining Form

dendr/o

Integumentary System

Combining Form

derm/a, derm/o, dermat/o

Combining Form

cyst/o, cyst/i

Urinary System

Gastrointestinal System

Prefix

Combining Form

Suffix

Combining Form

dactyl/o

General Terminology

Combining Form

Blood and the Immune System

Cardiovascular System

Endocrine System

Gastrointestinal System

General Terminology

Integumentary System

Gastrointestinal System

Combining Form

dent/o, dent/i

Musculoskeletal System

Nervous System and Mental Health

Reproductive Systems

Respiratory System

The Senses

Urinary System

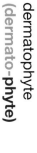

tears, lacrimal sac or duct

Word Building Example:

**dacryoadenitis
(dacryo-aden-itis)**

Inflammation of the lacrimal gland.

---

tree-shaped

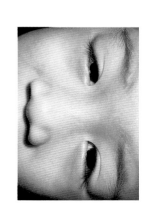

**bladder;
cystic duct**

Word Building Example:

**cystoscopy
(cysto-scopy)**

The inspection of the interior of the bladder by means of a cystoscope.

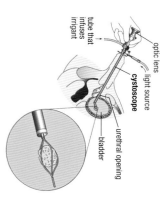

tube that
infuses
irrigant

optic lens

light source

cystoscope

urethral opening

bladder

---

digit (finger or toe)

Word Building Example:

**megadactyly
(mega-dactyl-y)**

Condition characterized by enlargement of one or more digits (fingers or toes).

---

skin

Word Building Example:

**dendriform
(dendri-form)**

Tree-shaped, or branching.

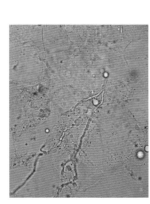

---

teeth, dental

Word Building Example:

**dentition
(denti-tion)**

The natural teeth, as considered collectively, in the dental arch; may be deciduous, permanent, or mixed.

permanent **dentition**

lower jaw

Word Building Example:

**dermatophyte
(dermato-phyte)**

A fungus that causes superficial infections of the skin, hair, and nails, i.e., keratinized tissues.

dextr/o

General Terminology

desm/o

Musculoskeletal System

Prefix

Combining Form

Suffix

dipl/o

Combining Form

The Senses

diaphor/o

Combining Form

General Terminology

Blood and the Immune System

Cardiovascular System

Endocrine System

Gastrointestinal System

General Terminology

Integumentary System

disc/o

Combining Form

Musculoskeletal System

dips/o

Combining Form

Endocrine System

Musculoskeletal System

Nervous System and Mental Health

Reproductive Systems

Respiratory System

The Senses

Urinary System

right

Word Building Example:
dextrogastria
(dextro-gastr-ia)

Condition in which the stomach is displaced to the right.

---

double, twofold

Word Building Example:
diplococcus
(diplo-coccus)

1. Spheric or ovoid bacterial cells joined together in pairs.
2. Common name of any organism belonging to the former bacterial genus *Diplococcus*.

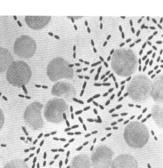

---

disk, disk-shaped

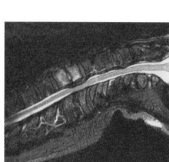

Word Building Example:
discectomy
(disc-ectomy)

Excision, in part or whole, of an intervertebral disc.

---

fibrous connection, ligament

Word Building Example:
desmitis
(desm-itis)

Inflammation of a ligament.

---

profuse sweating

Word Building Example:
diaphoretic
(diaphore-tic)

Relating to, or causing, perspiration.

---

thirst

Word Building Example:
polydipsia
(poly-dips-ia)

Excessive thirst that is relatively prolonged.

Card 428

Musculoskeletal System

dors/i, dors/o

Card 427

General Terminology

Combining Form

dist/o

Prefix

Combining Form

Suffix

Card 430

Combining Form

General Terminology

echin/o

Card 429

Combining Form

Gastrointestinal System

duoden/o

Blood and the Immune System

Cardiovascular System

Endocrine System

Gastrointestinal System

General Terminology

Integumentary System

Card 432

Combining Form

Blood and the Immune System

embol/o

Card 431

Combining Form

General Terminology

electr/o

Musculoskeletal System

Nervous System and Mental Health

Reproductive Systems

Respiratory System

The Senses

Urinary System

Word Building Example:

dorsiduct
(dorsi-duct)

To draw backward or toward the back.

prickly, spiny

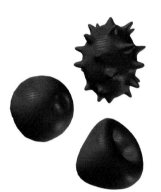

something inserted

Word Building Example:

echinocyte
(echino-cyte)

A crenated red blood cell.

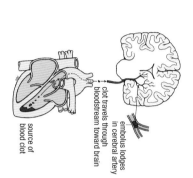

source of
blood clot

clot travels through
bloodstream toward brain

embolus lodges
in cerebral artery

Word Building Example:

embolism
(embol-ism)

Obstruction or occlusion of a vessel by an embolus.

Word Building Example:

distobuccal
(disto-bucc-al)

Relating to the distal and buccal surfaces of a tooth; denoting the angle formed by their junction.

duodenum

Word Building Example:

duodenum
(duoden-um)

The first division of the small intestine, about 25 cm or 12 fingerbreadths (hence the name) long, extending from the pylorus to the junction with the jejunum at the level of the first or second lumbar vertebra on the left side.

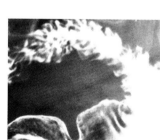

electricity

Word Building Example:

electroencephalography
(electro-encephalo-graphy)

Registration of the electrical potentials recorded by an electroencephalograph.

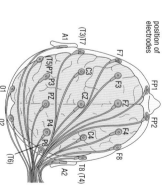

position of
electrodes

FP1
FP2
F7
F3
FZ
F4
F8
A1
(T3)T7
C3
CZ
C4
T8 (T4)
A2
(T5)P7
P3
PZ
P4
P8
(T6)
O1
O2

Card
433

Reproductive Systems

Prefix

Combining Form

Suffix

embry/o

Combining Form

Card
434

Nervous System & Mental Health

encephal/o

Combining Form

Card
435

Endocrine System

Blood and the Immune System

Cardiovascular System

Endocrine System

Gastrointestinal System

General Terminology

Integumentary System

endocrin/o

Combining Form

Card
436

Gastrointestinal System

enter/o

Combining Form

Card
437

Blood and the Immune System

Musculoskeletal System

Nervous System and Mental Health

Reproductive Systems

Respiratory System

The Senses

Urinary System

Urinary System

eosin/o

Combining Form

Card
438

epididym/o

Combining Form

brain

Word Building Example:

encephalomyelitis
(encephalo-myel-itis)

Inflammation of the brain and spinal cord.

small intestine

Word Building Example:

enterostomy
(entero-stomy)

An artificial anus or fistula into the intestine through the abdominal wall.

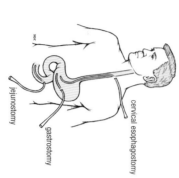

jejunostomy

gastrostomy

cervical esophagostomy

ser.

epididymis

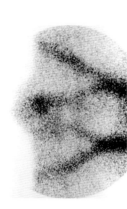

Word Building Example:

epididymitis
(epididym-itis)

Inflammation of the epididymis.

embryo

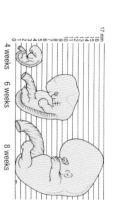

17 mm
16
15
14
13
12
11
10
9
8
7
6
5
4
3
2
1
0

4 weeks   6 weeks   8 weeks

Word Building Example:

embryogenesis
(embryo-genesis)

That phase of prenatal development involved in establishment of the characteristic configuration of the embryonic body.

endocrine

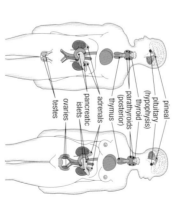

pineal
pituitary
(hypophysis)
thyroid
parathyroids
(posterior)
thymus
adrenals
pancreatic islets
ovaries
testes

Word Building Example:

endocrinology
(endocrino-logy)

The science and medical specialty concerned with the internal or hormonal secretions and their physiologic and pathologic relations.

rose-colored

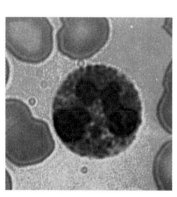

Word Building Example:

eosinophil
(eosino-phil)

A polymorphonuclear white blood cell characterized by prominent cytoplasmic granules that are bright yellow-red or orange when treated with Wright stain.

episi/o

Reproductive Systems
Urinary System

Combining Form

General Terminology

epipl/o

General Terminology

Prefix
Combining Form
Suffix

Combining Form

Gastrointestinal System

erg/o

Combining Form

Integumentary System

epitheli/o

Combining Form

Blood and the Immune System
Cardiovascular System
Endocrine System
Gastrointestinal System
General Terminology
Integumentary System

esophag/o

Combining Form

General Terminology
Blood and the Immune System

erythr/o

Combining Form

Musculoskeletal System
Nervous System and Mental Health
Reproductive Systems
Respiratory System
The Senses
Urinary System

episiotomy
(episio-tomy)

Word Building Example:

Surgical incision of the vulva to prevent laceration at the time of delivery or to facilitate vaginal surgery.

work

ergonomics
(ergo-nomics)

Word Building Example:

The science of workplace, tools, and equipment designed to reduce worker discomfort, strain, and fatigue and to prevent work-related injuries.

esophagus

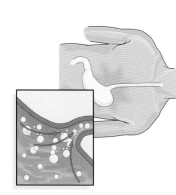

esophagitis
(esophag-itis)

Word Building Example:

Inflammation of the esophagus.

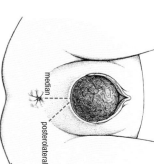
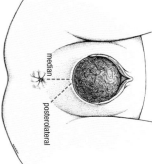

median

posterolateral

epiploon
(epiplo-on)

Word Building Example:

An areolar, four-layer peritoneal fold, formed by the double-layer dorsal mesentery of the stomach (dorsal mesogastrium) descending from the greater curvature of the stomach to fold under on itself and ascend to the transverse colon.

epithelium

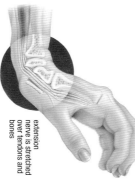
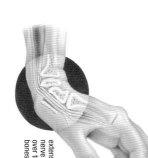

extension nerve is stretched over tendons and bones

epitheliolytic
(epithelio-lytic)

Word Building Example:

Destructive to epithelium.

denoting redness, red

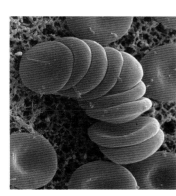

erythrocyte
(erythro-cyte)

Word Building Example:

A mature red blood cell.

Card
446

estr/o

Reproductive Systems
Endocrine System

Card
445

Combining Form

esthes/o, esthesi/o

Nervous System & Mental Health
The Senses

Prefix

Combining Form

Suffix

Card
448

eti/o

Combining Form

General Terminology

Card
447

Combining Form

Respiratory System

ethm/o

Blood and the Immune System

Cardiovascular System

Endocrine System

Gastrointestinal System

General Terminology

Integumentary System

Card
450

expir/o

Combining Form

Respiratory System

Card
449

Combining Form

Respiratory System

expector/o

Combining Form

Musculoskeletal System

Nervous System and Mental Health

Reproductive Systems

Respiratory System

The Senses

Urinary System

female

sensation

estrogen receptor
(estro-gen) receptor

Receptor for any substance, natural or synthetic, that exerts biologic effects characteristic of estrogenic hormones.

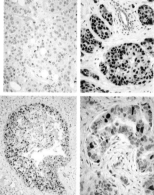
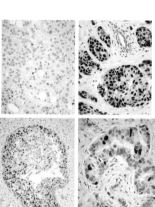

cause

esthesiometer
(esthesio-meter)

An instrument for determining the state of tactile and other forms of sensibility.

ethmoid

etiology
(etio-logy)

The science and study of the causes of disease and their mode of operation.

breath out

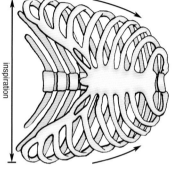

inspiration

ethmoidectomy
(ethm-oid-ectomy)

Removal of all or part of the mucosal lining and bony partitions between the ethmoid sinuses.

cough up

expiration
(expir-ation)

1. Breathing out. 2. Death.

expectorant
(expector-ant)

Promoting secretion from the mucous membrane of the air passages or facilitating its expulsion.

fasci/o

General Terminology
Musculoskeletal System

Combining Form

ferr/i, ferr/o

General Terminology
Blood and the Immune System

Combining Form

fibr/o

Musculoskeletal System

Combining Form

exud/o

Respiratory System

Prefix
Combining Form
Suffix

femor/o

Musculoskeletal System

Combining Form

Blood and the Immune System
Cardiovascular System
Endocrine System
Gastrointestinal System
General Terminology
Integumentary System

fet/o

Reproductive Systems

Combining Form

Musculoskeletal System
Nervous System and Mental Health
Reproductive Systems
Respiratory System
The Senses
Urinary System

fascia

Word Building Example:

fasciectomy
(fasci-ectomy)

Excision of strips of fascia.

---

iron

Word Building Example:

ferrokinetics
(ferro-kine-tics)

The study of iron metabolism using radioactive iron.

---

fiber

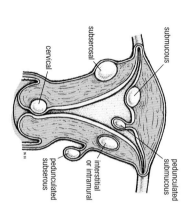

submucous

cervical

subserosal

pedunculated
subserous

interstitial
or intramural

pedunculated
submucous

---

fibroleiomyoma
(fibro-leio-my-oma)

A leiomyoma containing nonneoplastic collagenous fibrous tissue, which may make the tumor hard.

---

to sweat out

DESNOYERS
MANUS®

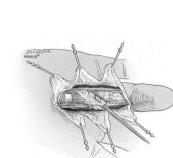

Word Building Example:

exudative retinitis
(exud-ative) retinitis

A chronic abnormality characterized by deposition of cholesterol and cholesterol esters in outer retinal layers and subretinal space.

---

femur

Word Building Example:

femoral artery
(femor-al) artery

Origin, continuation of external iliac, beginning at inguinal ligament; branches, external pudendal, superficial epigastric, superficial circumflex iliac, profunda femoris, descending genicular; terminating as the popliteal artery as it passes through the adductor hiatus to enter the popliteal space.

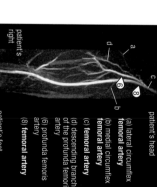

patient's
right

patient's head

(a) lateral circumflex
femoral artery

(b) medial circumflex
femoral artery

(c) **femoral artery**

(d) descending branch
of the profunda femoris
artery

(6) profunda femoris
artery

(8) **femoral artery**

patient's feet

---

fetus

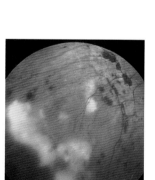

---

fetalism
(fet-al-ism)

Word Building Example:

Presence of certain fetal structures or characteristics in the body after birth.

flex/o

Musculoskeletal System

fibul/o

Musculoskeletal System

Prefix

Combining Form

Suffix

fluor/o

Combining Form

General Terminology

flu/o

Combining Form

General Terminology

Blood and the Immune System

Cardiovascular System

Endocrine System

Gastrointestinal System

General Terminology

Integumentary System

front/o

Combining Form

follicul/o

Integumentary System

Combining Form

Musculoskeletal System

Nervous System and Mental Health

Reproductive Systems

Respiratory System

The Senses

Urinary System

to bend

Word Building Example:
reflexophil
(re-flexo-phil)

Having exaggerated reflexes.

fibula

Word Building Example:
fibulocalcaneal
(fibulo-calcane-al)

Relating to the fibula and the calcaneus.

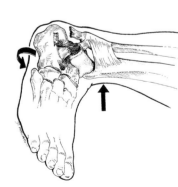

fluorine

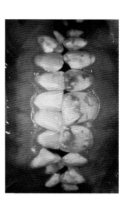

flow

Word Building Example:
fluorosis
(fluoro-sis)

A condition caused by an excessive intake of fluorides (2 or more ppm in drinking water), characterized mainly by mottling, staining, or hypoplasia of the enamel of the teeth, although the skeletal bones are also affected.

Word Building Example:
fluid
(flu-id)

A nonsolid substance that tends to flow or conform to the shape of the container in which it is kept.

forehead, brow

follicle

Word Building Example:
frontotemporal
(fronto-tempor-al)

Relating to the frontal and the temporal bones.

Word Building Example:
folliculosis
(follicul-osis)

Presence of lymph follicles in abnormally great numbers.

Card
464

galact/o

General Terminology

Combining Form

Card
463

fung/i

General Terminology

Prefix

Combining Form

Suffix

Combining Form

Card
466

gangli/o, ganglion/o

Nervous System & Mental Health

Combining Form

Card
465

gamet/o

Reproductive Systems

Combining Form

Blood and the Immune System

Cardiovascular System

Endocrine System

Gastrointestinal System

General Terminology

Integumentary System

Card
468

gen/o

General Terminology

Combining Form

Card
467

gastr/o

Gastrointestinal System

Combining Form

Musculoskeletal System

Nervous System and Mental Health

Reproductive Systems

Respiratory System

The Senses

Urinary System

milk

galactocele
(galacto-cele)

Retention cyst caused by occlusion of a lactiferous duct.

---

ganglion

---

being born, producing, coming to be

Word Building Example:

ganglioplegic
(ganglio-plegic)

A pharmacologic compound that paralyzes an autonomic ganglion, usually for a relatively short time.

Word Building Example:

genotype
(geno-type)

1. The genetic constitution of an individual. 2. Gene combination at one specific locus or any specified combination of loci.

---

fungus

Word Building Example:

fungiform
(fungi-form)

Shaped like a fungus or mushroom; applied to any structure with a broad, often branched, free portion and a narrower base.

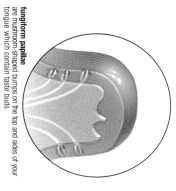

fungiform papillae
are mushroom-shaped bumps on the top and sides of your tongue which contain taste buds

---

wife or husband,
egg or sperm

Word Building Example:

gametocyte
(gameto-cyte)

A cell capable of dividing to produce gametes, e.g., a spermatocyte or oocyte.

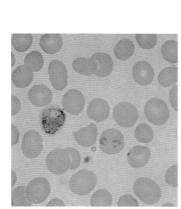

---

stomach, abdomen

Word Building Example:

gastroenterostomy
(gastro-entero-stomy)

Establishment of a new opening between the stomach and the intestine, either anterior or posterior to the transverse colon.

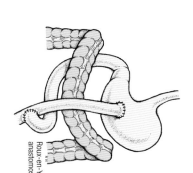

Roux-en-Y
anastomosis

gest/o

Reproductive Systems

ger/e, ger/o, geront/o

General Terminology

Prefix

Combining Form

Suffix

Combining Form

---

glauc/o

Combining Form

The Senses

gingiv/o

Combining Form

Gastrointestinal System

Blood and the Immune System

Cardiovascular System

Endocrine System

Gastrointestinal System

General Terminology

Integumentary System

---

glomerul/o

Combining Form

Combining Form

Urinary System

gli/o

Combining Form

Nervous System & Mental Health

Musculoskeletal System

Nervous System and Mental Health

Reproductive Systems

Respiratory System

The Senses

Urinary System

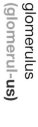

gestational sac (gest-ation-al) sac

Cystic structure of early pregnancy that represents the amniotic sac, fluid, and placenta.

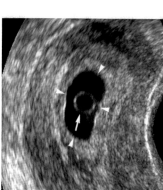

gray

glaucoma (glauc-oma)

Ocular disease associated with increased intraocular pressure and excavation and atrophy of the optic nerve; produces defects in the visual field and may result in blindness.

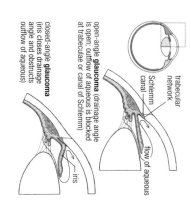

open-angle **glaucoma** (drainage angle is open; outflow of aqueous is blocked at trabecula or canal of Schlemm)

closed-angle **glaucoma** (iris closes drainage angle and obstructs outflow of aqueous)

trabecular network

Schlemm canal

flow of aqueous

iris

glomerulus (little ball)

glomerulus (glomerul-us)

1. A plexus of capillaries. 2. A tuft formed of capillary loops at the beginning of each nephric tubule in the kidney. 3. The twisted secretory portion of a sweat gland. 4. A cluster of dendritic ramifications and axon terminals forming a complex synaptic relationship and surrounded by a glial sheath.

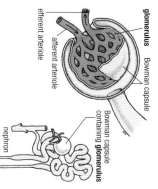

glomerulus

afferent arteriole

efferent arteriole

Bowman capsule

Bowman capsule containing **glomerulus**

nephron

---

geriatrics (ger-iatrics)

The branch of medicine concerned with the medical problems and care of old people.

gingivae, gums of the mouth

gingivitis (gingiv-itis)

Inflammation of the gingiva as a response to bacterial plaque on adjacent teeth; characterized by erythema, edema, and fibrous enlargement of the gingiva without resorption of the underlying alveolar bone.

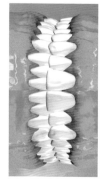

glue, glue-like (relating specifically to the neuroglia)

glioma (gli-oma)

Any neoplasm derived from one of the various types of cells that form the interstitial tissue of the brain, spinal cord, pineal gland, posterior pituitary gland, and retina.

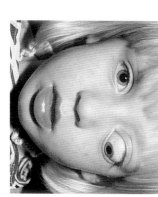

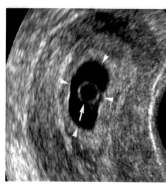

glott/o

Respiratory System

Combining Form

gloss/o

The Senses
Gastrointestinal System

Prefix

Combining Form

Suffix

---

glyc/o

Endocrine System

Combining Form

gluc/o, glucos/o

Endocrine System

Combining Form

Blood and the Immune System

Cardiovascular System

Endocrine System

Gastrointestinal System

General Terminology

Integumentary System

---

gnos/o

Combining Form

gnath/o

Nervous System & Mental Health

Musculoskeletal System

Combining Form

Musculoskeletal System

Nervous System and Mental Health

Reproductive Systems

Respiratory System

The Senses

Urinary System

opening

**glottitis
(glott-itis)**

Word Building Example:

Inflammation of the glottic portion of the larynx.

relating to sugars

**glycogenosis
(glyco-gen-osis)**

Word Building Example:

Any glycogen deposition disease characterized by accumulation of glycogen of normal or abnormal chemical structure in tissue.

knowledge

**gnosia
(gnos-ia)**

Word Building Example:

The perceptive faculty enabling one to recognize the form and the nature of people and things;

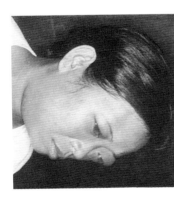

language (G. tongue)

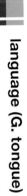

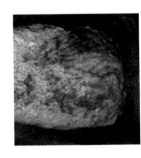

**glossotrichia
(glosso-trichia)**

Word Building Example:

A tongue with abnormal elongation of the filiform papillae, resulting in a thickened furry appearance.

relationship to glucose, sugar

**glucogenic
(gluco-genic)**

Word Building Example:

Giving rise to or producing glucose.

jaw

**gnathostomiasis
(gnatho-stom-iasis)**

Word Building Example:

A migrating edema, or creeping eruption, caused by cutaneous infection by larvae of *Gnathostoma spinigerum*.

Card 482

gonad/o

Reproductive Systems
Endocrine System

Card 484

granul/o

Combining Form
General Terminology

Card 486

halit/o

Combining Form

Card 481

gon/o

Reproductive Systems

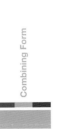

Prefix
Combining Form
Suffix

Card 483

goni/o

Combining Form
General Terminology

Blood and the Immune System
Cardiovascular System
Endocrine System
Gastrointestinal System
General Terminology
Integumentary System

Card 485

gyn/o, gynec/o

Reproductive Systems
Respiratory System
Combining Form

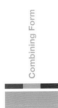

Musculoskeletal System
Nervous System and Mental Health
Reproductive Systems
Respiratory System
The Senses
Urinary System

gonads, sex glands

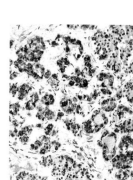

Word Building Example:

gonadotroph
(gonado-troph)

An endocrine cell of the adenohypophysis that affects certain cells of the ovary or testis.

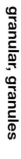

granular, granules

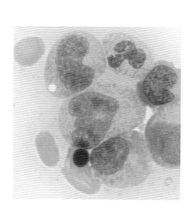

Word Building Example:

granulocytopenia
(granulo-cyto-penia)

Fewer than the normal number of granular leukocytes in the blood.

breath

Word Building Example:

halitosis
(halit-osis)

Foul mouth odor.

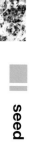

seed

Word Building Example:

gonococcus
(gono-coccus)

A bacterial species that causes gonorrhea and other infections in humans; the type species of the genus *Neisseria*.

angle

Word Building Example:

goniometer
(gonio-meter)

1. An instrument for measuring joint angles. 2. An appliance used in the static test of labyrinthine disease. 3. A calibrated device used to measure the arc or range of motion of a joint.

angle of 30°

female

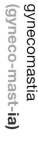

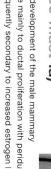

Word Building Example:

gynecomastia
(gyneco-mast-ia)

Excessive development of the male mammary glands, due mainly to ductal proliferation with periductal edema; frequently secondary to increased estrogen levels, but mild gynecomastia may occur in normal adolescence.

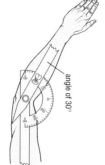

hedon/o

General Terminology

hallucin/o

Nervous System & Mental Health

Combining Form

Prefix

Combining Form

Suffix

hemangi/o

Combining Form

General Terminology
Blood and the Immune System

hem/o, hemat/o

Combining Form

General Terminology
Blood and the Immune System

Blood and the Immune System

Cardiovascular System

Endocrine System

Gastrointestinal System

General Terminology

Integumentary System

herni/o

Combining Form

Gastrointestinal System

hepat/o, hepatic/o

Combining Form

Gastrointestinal System

Musculoskeletal System

Nervous System and Mental Health

Reproductive Systems

Respiratory System

The Senses

Urinary System

pleasure

hedonophobia
(hedono-phobia)

Morbid fear of pleasure.

blood vessel

hernia, rupture, protrusion of a part of structure through the tissues containing it

Word Building Example:
hemangioma
(hemangi-oma)

A congenital anomaly in which proliferation of blood vessels leads to a mass that resembles a neoplasm.

Word Building Example:
herniotomy
(hernio-tomy)

Rupture of the liver.

to wander in the mind

Word Building Example:
hallucinogen
(hallucino-gen)

A mind-altering chemical, drug, or agent that elicits optic or auditory hallucinations, depersonalization, perceptual disturbances, and disturbances of thought processes.

blood

Word Building Example:
hematoma
(hemat-oma)

A localized mass of extravasated blood that is relatively or completely confined within an organ or tissue, a space, or a potential space.

liver

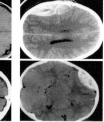
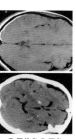

epidural (extradural) hemorrhages

acute subdural **hematoma** (left image) and subacute subdural **hematoma** (right image)

Word Building Example:
hepatocholangitis
(hepato-cholang-itis)

The crushing or fragmentation of a biliary calculus in the hepatic duct.

hist/o, histi/o

General Terminology

Musculoskeletal System

Combining Form

Musculoskeletal System

hidr/o

Integumentary System

Endocrine System

Combining Form

Prefix

Combining Form

Suffix

humer/o

Combining Form

Nervous System & Mental Health

Endocrine System

Combining Form

hormon/o

Blood and the Immune System

Cardiovascular System

Endocrine System

Gastrointestinal System

General Terminology

Integumentary System

hypn/o

Combining Form

General Terminology

Nervous System & Mental Health

Combining Form

hydr/o

Musculoskeletal System

Nervous System and Mental Health

Reproductive Systems

Respiratory System

The Senses

Urinary System

tissue, especially connective tissue

Word Building Example:

histiocyte
(histio-cyte)

A tissue macrophage; the class includes hepatic Kupffer cells, alveolar macrophages, giant cells of granulomas, osteoclasts, and dermal Langerhans cells. These cells derive from precursors that normally reside in bone marrow but migrate through the bloodstream to egress into tissues for final differentiation.

humerus

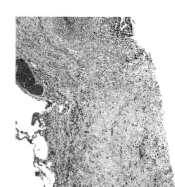

sweat glands

Word Building Example:

hidrocystoma
(hidro-cyst-oma)

A cystic form of neoplasm derived from epithelial cells of sweat glands.

Word Building Example:

humeroradial
(humero-radi-al)

Relating to both humerus and radius; denoting especially the ratio of length of one to the other.

sleep, hypnosis; sleep

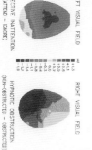

hormone

Word Building Example:

hormonogenic
(hormono-gen-ic)

Pertaining to the formation of a hormone.

water, watery; containing or combined with hydrogen

Word Building Example:

hypnosis
(hypn-osis)

An artificially induced trancelike state, resembling somnambulism, in which the subject is highly susceptible to suggestion and responds readily to the commands of the hypnotist.

Word Building Example:

hydrocele
(hydro-cele)

Collection of serous fluid in a sacculated cavity.

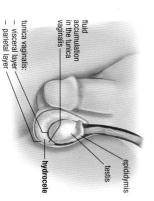

hyster/o

Reproductive Systems

hypophys/o

Endocrine System

Prefix

Combining Form

Suffix

ichthy/o

Combining Form

Integumentary System

iatr/o

Combining Form

General Terminology

Blood and the Immune System

Cardiovascular System

Endocrine System

Gastrointestinal System

General Terminology

Integumentary System

ide/o

Combining Form

icter/o

Combining Form

Nervous System & Mental Health

The Senses

Musculoskeletal System

Nervous System and Mental Health

Reproductive Systems

Respiratory System

The Senses

Urinary System

uterus, womb

Word Building Example:

hysterectomy
(hyster-ectomy)

Removal of the uterus; unless otherwise specified, usually denotes complete removal of the uterus.

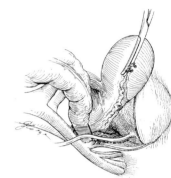

pituitary gland (hypophysis)

Word Building Example:

hypophysitis
(hypophys-itis)

Inflammation of the hypophysis.

fish, scaly, dry

Word Building Example:

ichthyosis
(ichthy-osis)

Congenital disorders of keratinization characterized by noninflammatory dryness and scaling of the skin, often associated with other defects and with abnormalities of lipid metabolism.

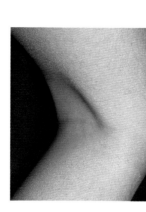

ideas, ideation

physicians, medicine, treatment

Word Building Example:

iatrogenic
(iatro-genic)

Denoting response to medical or surgical treatment, usually unfavorable.

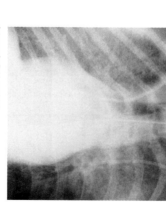

Iatrogenic fluid overload

icterus, jaundice

Word Building Example:

icterohemoglobinuria
(ictero-hemo-globin-uria)

Jaundice with hemoglobin in the urine.

Word Building Example:

idiomuscular
(idio-muscul-ar)

Relating to the muscles alone, independent of the nervous control.

ile/o

Gastrointestinal System

Combining Form

General Terminology

idi/o

General Terminology

Prefix

Combining Form

Suffix

immun/o

Combining Form

General Terminology

Combining Form

Musculoskeletal System

ili/o

Combining Form

Blood and the Immune System

Cardiovascular System

Endocrine System

Gastrointestinal System

General Terminology

Integumentary System

inguin/o

Combining Form

Gastrointestinal System

Urinary System

Combining Form

General Terminology

in/o

Combining Form

Musculoskeletal System

Nervous System and Mental Health

Reproductive Systems

Respiratory System

The Senses

Urinary System

ileum, groin, longest portion of the small intestine

Word Building Example:

ileostomy
(ileo-stomy)

Establishment of a fistula through which the ileum discharges the bowel's contents directly to the outside of the body. A type of fecal diversion.

immune, immunity, protection, resistant to an infectious disease

groin

Word Building Example:

immunoelectrophoresis
(immuno-electro-phoresis)

A kind of precipitin test in which the components of one group of immunologic reactants are first separated on the basis of electrophoretic mobility, the separated components then being identified on the basis of precipitates formed by reaction with components of the other group of reactants.

Word Building Example:

inguinoperitoneal
(inguino-periton-eal)

Relating to the groin and the peritoneum.

---

private, distinctive, peculiar, one's own

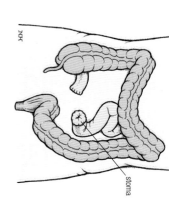

stoma

Word Building Example:

idiopathy
(idio-pathy)

A disease of unknown cause or mechanism.

ilium, broad portion of the hip bone

Word Building Example:

iliofemoroplasty
(ilio-femoro-plasty)

An obsolete method of securing a hip fusion by an extra-articular technique, a joint bypass procedure in which a turned down bone flap from the ilium is placed into a split in the greater trochanter.

fiber, muscle fiber

Word Building Example:

inotropic
(ino-tropic)

Influencing the contractility of muscular tissue.

iod/o

General Terminology

insul/o

Gastrointestinal System

Prefix

Combining Form

Suffix

---

ir/o, irit/o, irid/o

Combining Form

The Senses

ion/o

Combining Form

General Terminology

Blood and the Immune System

Cardiovascular System

Endocrine System

Gastrointestinal System

General Terminology

Integumentary System

---

jejun/o

Gastrointestinal System

Combining Form

ischi/o

Musculoskeletal System

Combining Form

Musculoskeletal System

Nervous System and Mental Health

Reproductive Systems

Respiratory System

The Senses

Urinary System

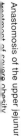

iodine

Word Building Example:

iododerma
(iodo-derma)

An eruption of follicular papules and pustules, or a granulomatous lesion, caused by iodine toxicity or sensitivity.

iris

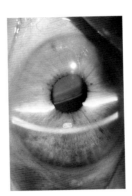

pancreatic islets

Word Building Example:

insulinoma
(insulin-oma)

An islet cell adenoma that secretes insulin.

ion

Word Building Example:

iridectomy
(irid-ectomy)

1. Excision of a portion of the iris. 2. The hole in the iris produced by a surgical iridectomy.

Word Building Example:

ionophore
(iono-phore)

A compound or substance that forms a complex with an ion and transports it across a membrane.

portion of small intestine between the duodenum and ileum;
jejunum, jejunal

ischium, hip joint, haunch

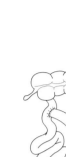

Word Building Example:

jejunoileal bypass
(jejuno-ile-al) bypass

Anastomosis of the upper jejunum to the terminal ileum for

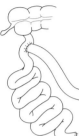

Word Building Example:

ischiocapsular
(ischio-capsul-ar)

Relating to the ischium and capsule of the hip joint; denoting that part of the capsule attached to the ischium.

kal/i

General Terminology

| Prefix |
| Combining Form |
| Suffix |

kary/o

General Terminology

kerat/o

Combining Form

The Senses | Integumentary System

| Blood and the Immune System |
| Cardiovascular System |
| Endocrine System |
| Gastrointestinal System |
| General Terminology |
| Integumentary System |

ket/o, keton/o

Combining Form

Urinary System

kin/o, kin/e,
kines/i, kinesi/o

Combining Form

General Terminology

| Musculoskeletal System |
| Nervous System and Mental Health |
| Reproductive Systems |
| Respiratory System |
| The Senses |
| Urinary System |

klepto/o

Combining Form

Nervous System & Mental Health

Word Building Example:

karyotype
(karyo-type)

The chromosome characteristics of an individual cell or of a cell line, usually presented as a systematized array of metaphase chromosomes from a photomicrograph of a single cell nucleus arranged in pairs in descending order of size and according to the position of the centromere.

ketone bodies

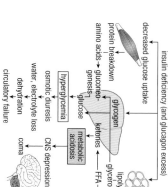

Word Building Example:

ketoacidosis
(keto-acid-osis)

Acidosis, due to enhanced production of ketone bodies.

to steal

Word Building Example:

kleptomania
(klepto-mania)

A disorder of impulse control characterized by a morbid tendency to steal.

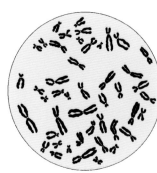

Word Building Example:

kaliopenia
(kalio-penia)

Insufficiency of potassium in the body.

cornea;
horny tissue or cells

Word Building Example:

keratoconus
(kerato-con-us)

A conic protrusion of the cornea caused by thinning of the stroma; usually bilateral.

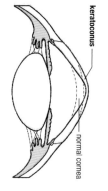

keratoconus —
— normal cornea

motion

Word Building Example:

kinetic
(kine-tic)

Relating to motion or movement.

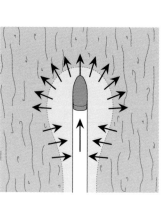

When a high-powered bullet enters the body, it transfers its **kinetic** energy to the surrounding tissues.

lips (also cheil/o-)

labial lesions
(labi-al) lesions

Lesions of any lip-shaped structures

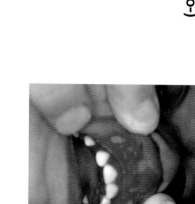

kyphosis
(kypho-tic)

1. An anteriorly concave curvature of the vertebral column.
2. Hyperkyphosis; excessive anteriorly concave curvature of a part of the spine.

hump

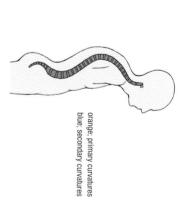

orange; primary curvatures
blue; secondary curvatures

---

tears

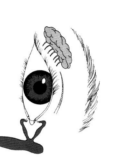

lacrimation
(lacrim-ation)

The secretion of tears, especially in excess.

labyrinth (inner ear)

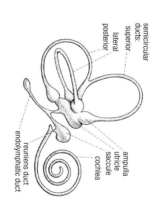

semicircular ducts:
superior
posterior
lateral

utricle
saccule
ampulla
cochlea

reuniens duct
endolymphatic duct

labyrinthitis
(labrinth-itis)

Inflammation of the labyrinth (the internal ear), sometimes accompanied by vertigo and deafness.

---

lamina

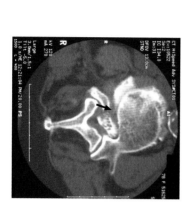

laminectomy
(lamin-ectomy)

Excision of a vertebral lamina; commonly used to denote removal of the posterior arch.

milk

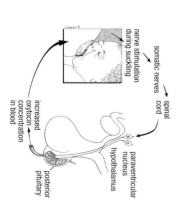

nerve stimulation
during suckling

somatic nerves

spinal cord

increased oxytocin concentration in blood

paraventricular nucleus

hypothalamus

posterior pituitary

lactation
(lact-ation)

1. Production of milk. 2. Period following birth during which milk is secreted in the breasts.

laryng/o

The Senses

lapar/o

General Terminology
Gastrointestinal System

Prefix
Combining Form
Suffix

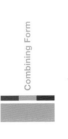

---

lei/o

Combining Form

General Terminology

later/o

Combining Form

General Terminology

Blood and the Immune System
Cardiovascular System
Endocrine System
Gastrointestinal System
General Terminology
Integumentary System

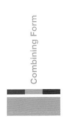

---

lept/o

Combining Form

lent/i

Combining Form

The Senses

Musculoskeletal System
Nervous System and Mental Health
Reproductive Systems
Respiratory System
The Senses
Urinary System

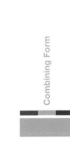

larynx

Word Building Example:

laryngospasm
(laryngo-spasm)

Spasmodic closure of the glottic aperture.

smooth

Word Building Example:

leiomyoma
(leio-my-oma)

A benign neoplasm derived from smooth (nonstriated) muscle.

light, thin, frail

Word Building Example:

leptomeningitis
(lepto-mening-itis)

Inflammation of two delicate layers of the meninges, the arachnoid mater and pia mater.

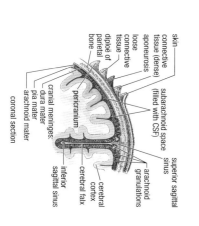

skin
connective tissue (dense)
aponeurosis
loose connective tissue
diploë of parietal bone

cranial meninges:
dura mater
pia mater
arachnoid mater
coronal section

pericranium

subarachnoid space (filled with CSF)

superior sagittal sinus

arachnoid granulations

cerebral falx
cerebral cortex
inferior sagittal sinus

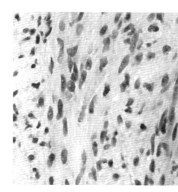

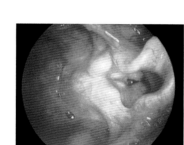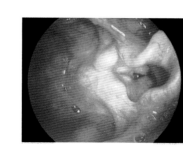

loins (less properly, the abdomen in general)

Word Building Example:

laparoscopy
(laparo-scopy)

Examination of the contents of the peritoneum with a laparoscope.

lateral, to one side

Word Building Example:

lateroflexion
(latero-flexion)

A bending or curvature to one side.

lens

Word Building Example:

lenticonus
(lenti-con-us)

Conical projection of the anterior or posterior surface of the lens of the eye, occurring as a developmental anomaly.

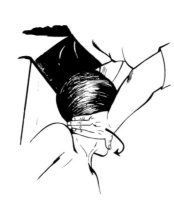

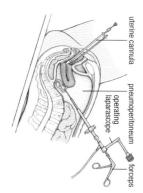

uterine cannula

operating laparoscope

pneumoperitoneum

forceps

lev/o

General Terminology

leuk/o, leuc/o

General Terminology

Blood and the Immune System

Prefix

Combining Form

Suffix

lingu/o

Combining Form

Gastrointestinal System

The Senses

lex/o

The Senses

Nervous System & Mental Health

Blood and the Immune System

Cardiovascular System

Endocrine System

Gastrointestinal System

General Terminology

Integumentary System

lith/o

Combining Form

Urinary System

lip/o

Combining Form

General Terminology

Integumentary System

Musculoskeletal System

Nervous System and Mental Health

Reproductive Systems

Respiratory System

The Senses

Urinary System

left, toward or on the left side

Word Building Example:

levoduction
(levo-duct-ion)

Turning of one eye to the left.

tongue

---

stone, calculus, calcification

Word Building Example:

linguopapillitis
(linguo-papill-itis)

Small, painful ulcers involving the papillae on the tongue margins.

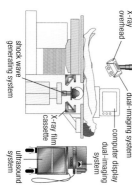

X-ray overhead

dual-imaging system

shock wave generating system

computer display dual-imaging system

X-ray film cassette

ultrasound system

Word Building Example:

lithotripsy
(litho-tripsy)

The crushing of a stone in the renal pelvis, ureter, or bladder, by mechanical force or sound waves.

---

white, white blood cells

Word Building Example:

leukocyte
(leuko-cyte)

A type of cell formed in the myelopoietic, lymphoid, and reticular portions of the reticuloendothelial system in various parts of the body, and normally present in those sites and in the circulating blood.

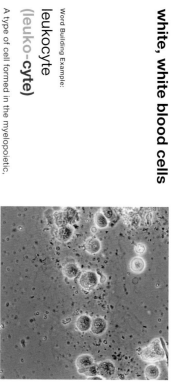

word or phrase

Word Building Example:

alexia
(a-lex-ia)

An inability to comprehend the meaning of written or printed words and sentences, caused by a cerebral lesion.

---

fatty, lipid

Word Building Example:

lipoma
(lip-oma)

A benign neoplasm of adipose tissue, composed of mature fat cells.

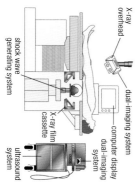

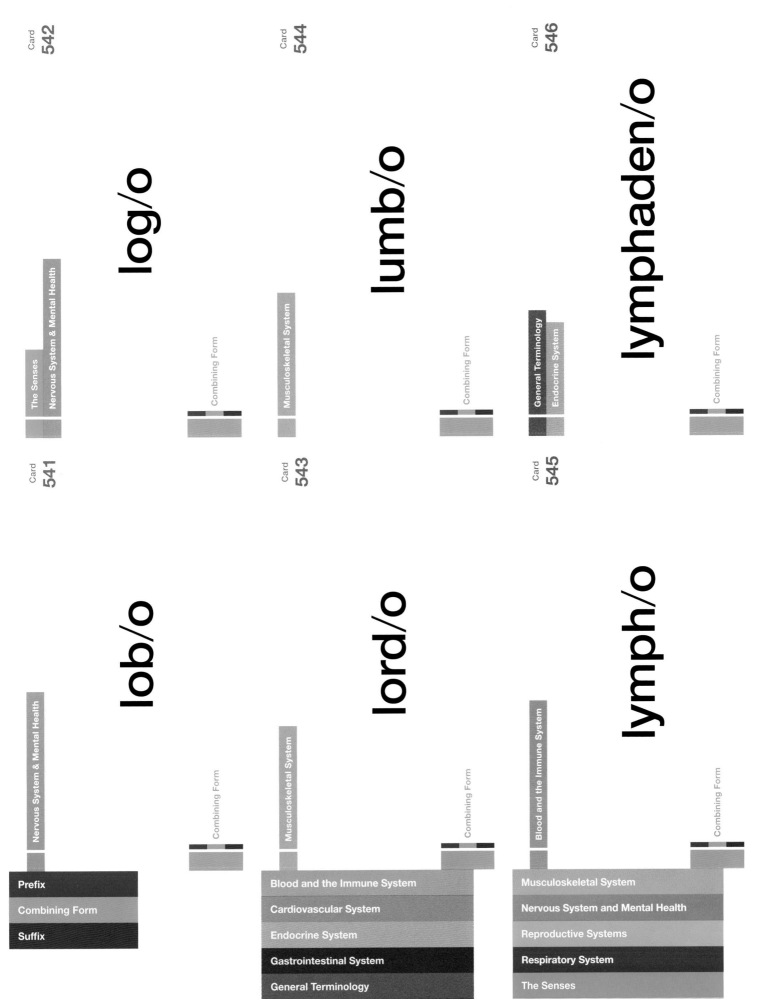

Card 542

log/o

The Senses

Nervous System & Mental Health

Combining Form

Card 541

lob/o

Nervous System & Mental Health

Prefix

Combining Form

Suffix

Card 544

lumb/o

Musculoskeletal System

Combining Form

Card 543

lord/o

Musculoskeletal System

Combining Form

Blood and the Immune System

Cardiovascular System

Endocrine System

Gastrointestinal System

General Terminology

Integumentary System

Card 546

lymphaden/o

General Terminology

Endocrine System

Combining Form

Card 545

lymph/o

Blood and the Immune System

Combining Form

Musculoskeletal System

Nervous System and Mental Health

Reproductive Systems

Respiratory System

The Senses

Urinary System

speech, words

Word Building Example:

logorrhea
(logo-rrhea)

Uncommon term for abnormal or pathologic talkativeness or garrulousness.

---

lumbar region, lower back

Word Building Example:

lumbosacral
(lumbo-sacr-al)

Relating to the lumbar vertebrae and the sacrum.

---

lymph nodes

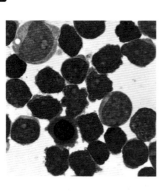

Word Building Example:

lymphadenography
(lymphadeno-graphy)

Radiographic visualization of lymph nodes after injection of a contrast medium.

---

lobe

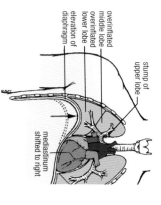

Word Building Example:

lobectomy
(lob-ectomy)

Excision of a lobe of any organ or gland.

---

curved, bent

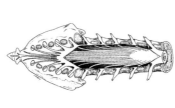

Word Building Example:

lordosis
(lord-osis)

An anteriorly convex curvature of the vertebral column.

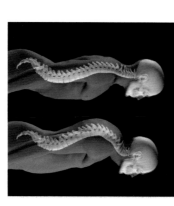

---

lymph

Word Building Example:

lymphoblastic leukemia
(lympho-blast-ic) leukemia

Acute lymphocytic leukemia in which the abnormal cells are chiefly (or almost totally) blast forms of the lymphocytic series, or in which unusually large numbers of the immature forms occur in association with adult lymphocytes.

mamm/o

Reproductive Systems
Endocrine System

lymphangi/o

General Terminology
Endocrine System

Combining Form

Prefix

Combining Form

Suffix

mast/o

Combining Form

Reproductive Systems
Gastrointestinal System

mandibul/o

Combining Form

Musculoskeletal System
The Senses

Combining Form

Blood and the Immune System

Cardiovascular System

Endocrine System

Gastrointestinal System

General Terminology

Integumentary System

meat/o

Combining Form

Combining Form

maxill/o

General Terminology

Musculoskeletal System
The Senses

Combining Form

Musculoskeletal System

Nervous System and Mental Health

Reproductive Systems

Respiratory System

The Senses

Urinary System

breast

mammogram
(mammo-gram)

The record produced by mammography.

---

breast; mastoid

digastric (anterior)
digastric (posterior)
stylohyoid
thyrohyoid
omohyoid (superior)
sternothyoid
omohyoid (inferior)
mylohyoid
hyoid bone
anterior scalene
sternocleido-mastoid
omohyoid
trapezius
subclavius

---

passage or channel, especially the external opening of a canal

---

mastication
(masti-cation)

The process of chewing food in preparation for deglutition and digestion; the act of grinding or comminuting with the teeth.

meatoplasty
(meato-plasty)

Enlargement or other surgical reconfiguring of a meatus or canal.

---

lymphatic vessels

lymphography
(lympho-graphy)

Visualization of lymphatics, lymph nodes, or both by radiography after intralymphatic injection of a contrast medium.

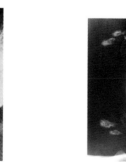

---

lower jaw

---

mandibulofacial dysostosis
(mandibulo-faci-al) dysostosis

A variable syndrome of malformations primarily of derivatives of the first pharyngeal arch.

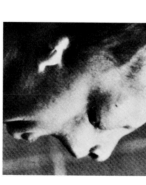

---

upper jaw

---

maxillomandibular
(maxillo-mandibul-ar)

Relating to the upper and lower jaws.

melan/o

General Terminology

Integumentary System

medull/o

General Terminology

Combining Form

Prefix

Combining Form

Suffix

mening/o,
meningi/o

Combining Form

Nervous System & Mental Health

men/o, mens

Combining Form

Reproductive Systems

Blood and the Immune System

Cardiovascular System

Endocrine System

Gastrointestinal System

General Terminology

Integumentary System

metabol/o

Combining Form

General Terminology

Gastrointestinal System

ment/o

Combining Form

Nervous System & Mental Health

Musculoskeletal System

Nervous System and Mental Health

Reproductive Systems

Respiratory System

The Senses

Urinary System

black, dark, melanin

Word Building Example:

melanoma
(melan-oma)

A malignant neoplasm, derived from cells that are capable of forming melanin.

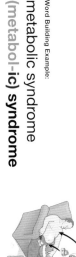

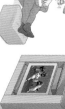

---

any membrane,
specifically, one of
the membranous
coverings of the brain
and spinal cord

Word Building Example:

meningitis
(mening-itis)

Inflammation of the membranes of the brain or spinal cord.

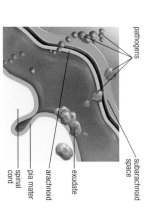

pathogens

subarachnoid
space

exudate

arachnoid

pia mater

spinal
cord

---

change

high blood pressure
• >140/90 mm Hg

blood abnormalities
• high blood glucose (fasting >110 mg/dL)
• high triglycerides (>150 mg/dL)
• low HDL cholesterol – males, <40 mg/dL – females, <50 mg/dL

waist
– males > 40" – females > 35"

Word Building Example:

metabolic syndrome
(metabol-ic) syndrome

The metabolic syndrome comprises several abnormalities, each an independent risk factor for cardiovascular disease, which have been associated on the premise of a unitary cause.

---

soft marrow-like structure,
especially in the center of a part

Word Building Example:

medulloblastoma
(medullo-blast-oma)

A tumor consisting of neoplastic cells that resemble the undifferentiated cells of the primitive medullary tube; usually located in the vermis of the cerebellum.

---

menses, menstruation

Word Building Example:

menopause
(meno-pause)

Permanent cessation of the menses.

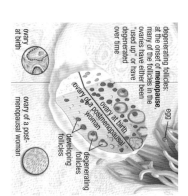

degenerating follicles:
at the onset of **menopause,**
many of the follicles in the
ovaries have either been
"used up" or have
degenerated
over time

ovary
at birth

ovary at birth

ovary of a postmenopausal
woman

ovary of a post-
menopausal woman

egg

developing
follicles

degenerating
follicles

---

the mind, mental,
psychologic; chin

Word Building Example:

dementia
(de-ment-ia)

The loss, usually progressive, of cognitive and intellectual functions, without impairment of perception or consciousness.

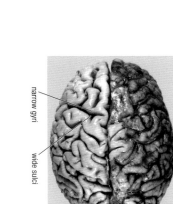

narrow gyri

wide sulci

Card
560

metatars/o

Musculoskeletal System

Card
562

Combining Form

General Terminology

morph/o

Combining Form

Card
564

Musculoskeletal System

muscul/o

Combining Form

Card
559

metacarp/o

Musculoskeletal System

Combining Form

Prefix

Combining Form

Suffix

Card
561

Reproductive Systems

metr/a, metr/o, metri/o

Combining Form

Blood and the Immune System

Cardiovascular System

Endocrine System

Gastrointestinal System

General Terminology

Integumentary System

Card
563

General Terminology

muc/i, muc/o

Combining Form

Musculoskeletal System

Nervous System and Mental Health

Reproductive Systems

Respiratory System

The Senses

Urinary System

metatarsus, bones of the foot

metatarsalgia
(metatars-algia)

Pain in the forefoot near the metatarsal heads.

---

form, structure

---

muscle

Science concerned with the structure of animals and plants.

morphology
(morpho-logy)

---

muscle

musculotendinous cuff
(musculo-tendin-ous) cuff

The anterior, superior, and posterior aspects of the capsule of the shoulder joint reinforced by the tendons of insertion of the supraspinatus, infraspinatus, teres minor, and subscapularis (SITS) muscles.

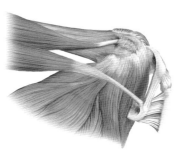

---

metacarpus, bones of the hand

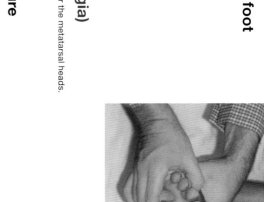

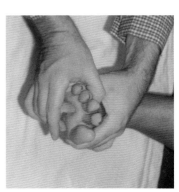

proximal interphalangeal joint
metacarpophalangeal joint
extensor digitorum tendon
interosseous muscle

lumbrical
"hood" anchoring expansion to palmar ligament
flexor digitorum superficialis tendon

median band
distal inter-phalangeal joint
distal phalanx
middle phalanx
flexor digitorum profundus tendon
lateral band
extensor expansion

metacarpophalangeal joints
(metacarpo-phalang-eal) joints

The condylar or ellipsoid synovial joints between the heads of the metacarpals and the bases of the proximal phalanges.

---

uterus

---

metrostenosis
(metro-sten-osis)

A narrowing of the uterine cavity.

**mucus, mucin
(also myx/o)**

**mucocele
(muco-cele)**

A retention cyst of the salivary gland, lacrimal sac, paranasal sinuses, appendix, or gallbladder.

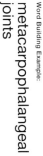
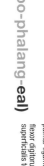

my/o, myos/o

Musculoskeletal System

mut/a

General Terminology

Prefix

Combining Form

Suffix

myel/o

Combining Form

Nervous System & Mental Health

Musculoskeletal System

myc/o

Combining Form

General Terminology

Blood and the Immune System

Cardiovascular System

Endocrine System

Gastrointestinal System

General Terminology

Integumentary System

myx/o

Combining Form

General Terminology

myring/o

Combining Form

The Senses

Musculoskeletal System

Nervous System and Mental Health

Reproductive Systems

Respiratory System

The Senses

Urinary System

muscle

Word Building Example:
myomectomy
(myom-ectomy)

Operative removal of a myoma, specifically of a uterine myoma.

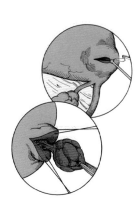

to change

Word Building Example:
mutagenesis
(muta-genesis)

1. Production of a mutation. 2. Production of genetic alteration through use of chemicals or radiation.

---

bone marrow;
spinal cord and
medulla oblongata

Word Building Example:
myelodysplasia
(myelo-dys-plasia)

1. An abnormality in development of the spinal cord, especially the lower part. 2. Bone marrow disorder, characterized by proliferation of abnormal stem cells, which have the potential of developing into leukemia.

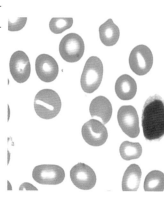

fungus

Word Building Example:
mycology
(myco-logy)

The study of fungi including pathogenicity.

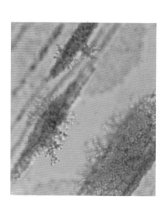

---

mucus

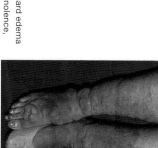
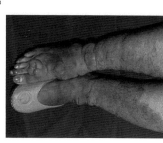

tympanic membrane

Word Building Example:
myxedema
(myx-edema)

Hypothyroidism characterized by a relatively hard edema of subcutaneous tissue; characterized by somnolence, slow mentation, dryness and loss of hair, increased fluid in body cavities, subnormal temperature, hoarseness, muscle weakness, and slow return of a muscle to the neutral position after a tendon jerk.

Word Building Example:
myringodermatitis
(myringo-dermat-itis)

Inflammation of the meatal or outer surface of the drum membrane and the adjoining skin of the external auditory canal.

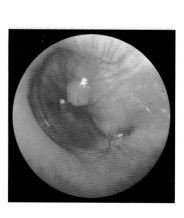

nas/o

The Senses

Combining Form

General Terminology

natr/i

Combining Form

General Terminology

nemat/o

Combining Form

narc/o

Nervous System & Mental Health

Prefix

Combining Form

Suffix

Combining Form

nat/a

Reproductive Systems

Combining Form

Blood and the Immune System

Cardiovascular System

Endocrine System

Gastrointestinal System

General Terminology

Integumentary System

necr/o

General Terminology

Integumentary System

Combining Form

Musculoskeletal System

Nervous System and Mental Health

Reproductive Systems

Respiratory System

The Senses

Urinary System

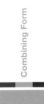
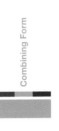

nose

nasopharynx
(naso-pharynx)

The part of the pharynx that lies above the soft palate; anteriorly it opens into the nasal cavity.

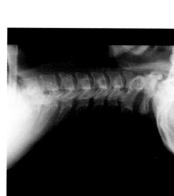

sodium

stupor, narcosis, numbness, sleep

narcotherapy
(narco-therapy)

Psychotherapy conducted with the patient under the influence of a sedative or narcotic.

birth

natremia
(natr-emia)

The presence of sodium in the blood.

thread, threadlike

intestinal villus
mouth
intestinal muscle

hookworm

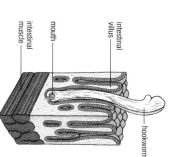
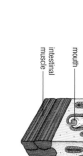

nematode
(nemat-ode)

A common name for any roundworm of the phylum Nematoda.

death, necrosis

natality
(nata-lity)

The birth rate; the ratio of births to the general population.

necrosis
(necr-osis)

Pathologic death of one or more cells, or of a portion of tissue or organ, resulting from irreversible damage.

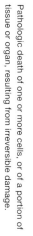

Card 577

nephr/o

Urinary System

Combining Form

Prefix
Combining Form
Suffix

Card 578

neur/o, neur/i

Nervous System & Mental Health
Endocrine System

Combining Form

Card 579

neutr/o

Blood and the Immune System

Combining Form

Blood and the Immune System
Cardiovascular System
Endocrine System
Gastrointestinal System
General Terminology
Integumentary System

Card 580

noct/u, nyct/o

General Terminology

Combining Form

Card 581

nos/o

General Terminology
Blood and the Immune System

Combining Form

Musculoskeletal System
Nervous System and Mental Health
Reproductive Systems
Respiratory System
The Senses
Urinary System

Card 582

nucle/o

Combining Form

neuroglia
(neuro-glia)

Nonneuronal cellular elements of the central and peripheral nervous system.

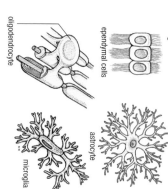

neuroglia

ependymal cells

oligodendrocyte

astrocyte

microglia

night

nocturia
(noct-uria)

Frequent urination at night.

nucleus

nuclear envelope
(nucle-ar) envelope

The double membrane at the boundary of the nucleoplasm; it has regularly spaced pores covered by a disc-like nuclear pore complex and a space or cisterna about 150 Å wide between the two membranes; the outer membrane is continuous at intervals with the rough endoplasmic reticulum.

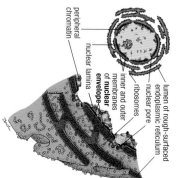

peripheral
chromatin

nuclear lamina

inner and outer
membranes
of **nuclear
envelope**

ribosomes

nuclear pore

lumen of rough-surfaced
endoplasmic reticulum

kidney

nephrolithiasis
(nephro-lith-iasis)

Presence of renal calculi, a calculus occurring within the kidney collecting system.

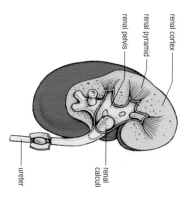

renal cortex

renal pyramid

renal pelvis

ureter

renal
calculi

neither

neutrophil
(neutro-phil)

A mature white blood cell in the granulocytic series, formed by myelopoietic tissue of the bone marrow (sometimes also in extramedullary sites) and released into the circulating blood, where they normally represent 54%–65% of the total number of leukocytes.

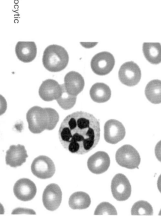

disease

nosoacusis
(noso-acusis)

Hearing loss due to disease, as opposed to aging.

occipit/o

Musculoskeletal System
Nervous System & Mental Health

obstetr/o

Reproductive Systems

Prefix

Combining Form

Suffix

odont/o

Combining Form

Gastrointestinal System

ocul/o

Combining Form

The Senses

Blood and the Immune System

Cardiovascular System

Endocrine System

Gastrointestinal System

General Terminology

Integumentary System

olecran/o

Combining Form

Musculoskeletal System

odyn/o

Combining Form

General Terminology

Musculoskeletal System

Nervous System and Mental Health

Reproductive Systems

Respiratory System

The Senses

Urinary System

occiput, occipital structures (back of the head)

Word Building Example:
occipitis
(occip-itis)

The back of the head.

midwife

Word Building Example:
obstetric forceps
(obstetr-ic) forceps

Forceps used for grasping and applying traction to or for rotation of the fetal head.

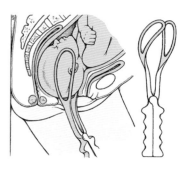

tooth, teeth

the eye, ocular

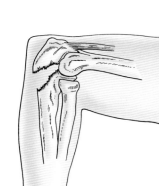

odontolysis (odonto-lysis)

Word Building Example:

Chemically induced tooth loss, occurring mainly through acid dissolution. When the cause is unknown, it is referred to as idiopathic erosion.

the head or point of the elbow

Word Building Example:
oculocutaneous albinism
(oculo-cutane-ous) albinism

A disorder characterized by deficiency of pigment in skin, hair, and eyes, causing photophobia, nystagmus, and decreased visual acuity.

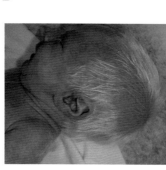

pain

Word Building Example:
olecranon fracture
(olecran-on) fracture

Fracture of the elbow bone.

Word Building Example:
odynophonia
(odyno-phonia)

Pain on using the voice.

olig/o

General Terminology

olfact/o

The Senses

Prefix

Combining Form

Suffix

---

oment/o

Combining Form

Gastrointestinal System

om/o

Musculoskeletal System

Combining Form

Blood and the Immune System

Cardiovascular System

Endocrine System

Gastrointestinal System

General Terminology

Integumentary System

---

onc/o, onch/o, onk/o

Combining Form

General Terminology

omphal/o

Gastrointestinal System
Reproductive Systems

Combining Form

Musculoskeletal System

Nervous System and Mental Health

Reproductive Systems

Respiratory System

The Senses

Urinary System

oligodendroglioma

Word Building Example:

(oligo-dendro-gli-oma)

A rare, slowly growing glioma derived from oligodendrocytes that occurs most frequently in the cerebrum of adults.

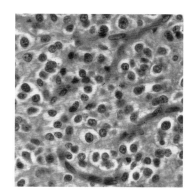

smell

Word Building Example:

olfaction

(olfact-ion)

The sense of smell.

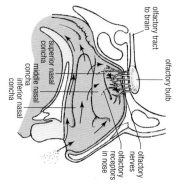

olfactory tract to brain

olfactory bulb

superior nasal concha
middle nasal concha
inferior nasal concha

olfactory nerves

olfactory receptors in nose

omentum

Word Building Example:

omentum

(oment-um)

A fold of peritoneum passing from the stomach to another abdominal organ.

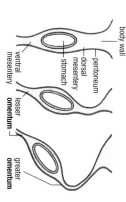

body wall
peritoneum
dorsal mesentery
stomach
ventral mesentery
lesser **omentum**
greater **omentum**

shoulder

Word Building Example:

omohyoid

(omo-hyoid)

Infrahyoid muscle; formed of two bellies attached to intermediate tendon; origin, by inferior belly from upper border of scapula between superior angle and notch; insertion, by superior belly into hyoid bone; action, depresses hyoid; nerve supply, upper cervical spinal nerves through ansa cervicalis.

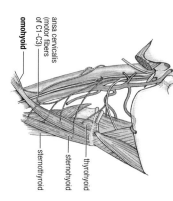

ansa cervicalis (motor fibers of C1–C3)

omohyoid

sternothyroid
sternohyoid
thyrohyoid

tumor, mass

Word Building Example:

oncosphere

(onco-sphere)

The motile six-hooked first-stage larva of cyclophyllidean cestodes; it emerges from the egg and actively claws its way through the intermediate host's intestine before development into the next larval stage.

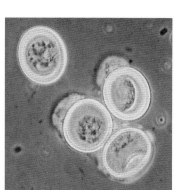

the umbilicus, the navel

Word Building Example:

omphalopagus

(omphalo-pagus)

Conjoined twins united at their umbilical regions.

onych/o

Prefix

Combining Form

Suffix

Integumentary System

oophor/o

Reproductive Systems

Combining Form

ophthalm/o

The Senses

Blood and the Immune System

Cardiovascular System

Endocrine System

Gastrointestinal System

General Terminology

Integumentary System

Combining Form

opisth/o

General Terminology

Combining Form

or/o

Respiratory System

The Senses

Musculoskeletal System

Nervous System and Mental Health

Reproductive Systems

Respiratory System

The Senses

Urinary System

Combining Form

orch/i, orchi/o, orchid/o

Reproductive Systems

Combining Form

ovary

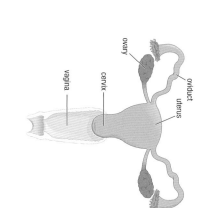

ovary · oviduct · uterus · cervix · vagina

Word Building Example:

oophorectomy
(oophor-ectomy)

Excision of one or both ovaries.

---

backward, behind, dorsal

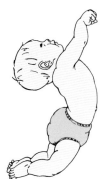

Word Building Example:

opisthotonos
(opistho-ton-os)

A tetanic spasm in which the spine and extremities are bent with convexity forward, the body resting on the head and the heels.

---

testes

Word Building Example:

orchidectomy
(orchid-ectomy)

Removal of one or both testes.

---

fingernail, toenail

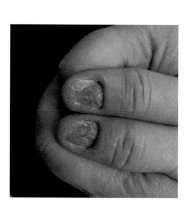

Word Building Example:

onychodystrophy
(onycho-dys-trophy)

Dystrophic changes in the nails occurring as a congenital defect or due to any illness or injury that may cause a malformed nail.

---

relationship to the eye

Word Building Example:

ophthalmoscopy
(ophthalmo-scopy)

Examination of the fundus of the eye by means of the ophthalmoscope.

---

mouth

posterior wall of **oropharynx**
soft palate
uvula
palatine tonsil
palatoglossal arch
palatopharyngeal arch
dorsum of tongue

Word Building Example:

oropharynx
(oro-pharynx)

The portion of the pharynx that lies posterior to the mouth; it is continuous above with the nasopharynx through the pharyngeal isthmus and below with the laryngopharynx.

Card 601

organ/o

General Terminology

Prefix
Combining Form
Suffix

Combining Form

Card 602

orth/o

General Terminology
Musculoskeletal System

Combining Form

Card 603

osche/o

Reproductive Systems

Blood and the Immune System
Cardiovascular System
Endocrine System
Gastrointestinal System
General Terminology
Integumentary System

Combining Form

Card 604

osm/o

General Terminology
The Senses

Combining Form

Card 605

osphresi/o

The Senses

Musculoskeletal System
Nervous System and Mental Health
Reproductive Systems
Respiratory System
The Senses
Urinary System

Combining Form

Card 606

oss/i, osse/o, oste/o

Musculoskeletal System

Combining Form

straight or normal,
in proper order

Word Building Example:

orthokeratology
(ortho-kerato-logy)

A method of molding the cornea with contact lenses to improve unaided vision.

---

osmosis;
smell, odor

Word Building Example:

osmology
(osmo-logy)

The study of odors, their production, and their effects.

---

bone, bony

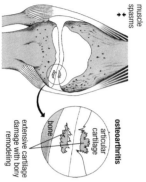

muscle
spasms

osteoarthritis
articular
cartilage
bone

extensive cartilage
damage with bony
remodeling

Word Building Example:

osteoarthritis
(osteo-arthr-itis)

Arthritis characterized by erosion of articular cartilage, either primary or secondary to trauma or other conditions, which becomes soft, frayed, and thinned with eburnation of subchondral bone and outgrowths of marginal osteophytes.

---

organ, organic

Word Building Example:

organogenesis
(organo-genesis)

Formation of organs during development.

---

scrotum

Word Building Example:

oscheohydrocele
(oscheo-hydro-cele)

Scrotal hydrocele.

---

odor;
sense of smell

Word Building Example:

osphresis
(osphres-is)

The sense of smell.

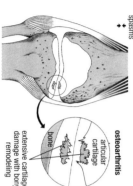

ov/i, ov/o, ovul/o

Reproductive Systems

ot/o

The Senses

Prefix

Combining Form

Suffix

ox/a, ox/o

Combining Form

General Terminology

ovari/o

Combining Form

Reproductive Systems

Blood and the Immune System

Cardiovascular System

Endocrine System

Gastrointestinal System

General Terminology

Integumentary System

palpebr/o

Combining Form

palat/o

Combining Form

The Senses

Gastrointestinal System

Musculoskeletal System

Nervous System and Mental Health

Reproductive Systems

Respiratory System

The Senses

Urinary System

egg

ear

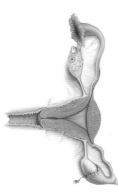

oviduct
(ovi-duct)

One of the tubes leading on either side from the upper or outer extremity of the ovary, which is largely enveloped by its expanded infundibulum, to the fundus of the uterus.

otomycosis
(oto-myc-osis)

Word Building Example:

Fungal infection in the external auditory canal, with scaling, itching, and pain as the primary symptoms.

oxygen

superior vena cava

right atrium

inferior vena cava

right endocardial cushion

superior vena cava

septum secundum

right ventricle

muscular ventricular septum

septum secundum

septum primum

left atrium

inferior endocardial cushion

left endocardial cushion

ventricle

septum primum

ostium secundum

foramen ovale

inferior endocardial cushion

left ventricle

ovary

ovarian cycle
(ovari-an) cycle

Word Building Example:

The normal sex cycle that includes development of an ovarian follicle, rupture of the follicle with discharge of the oocyte or ovum, and formation and regression of a corpus luteum.

oxygenate
(oxy-gen-ate)

Word Building Example:

To accomplish oxygenation.

eyelid

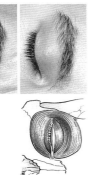

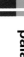

palate

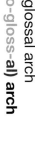

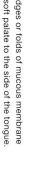

palpebrate
(palpebr-ate)

Word Building Example:

1. Having eyelids. 2. To wink.

palatoglossal arch
(palato-gloss-al) arch

Word Building Example:

One of a pair of ridges or folds of mucous membrane passing from the soft palate to the side of the tongue.

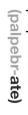

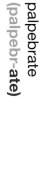

pant/o

General Terminology

Gastrointestinal System

pancre/o,
pancreat/o

Prefix

Combining Form

Suffix

Combining Form

Integumentary System

papul/o

Combining Form

General Terminology

The Senses

papill/o

Combining Form

Blood and the Immune System

Cardiovascular System

Endocrine System

Gastrointestinal System

General Terminology

Integumentary System

General Terminology

pariet/o

Combining Form

Endocrine System

parathyr/o,
parathyroid/o

Combining Form

Musculoskeletal System

Nervous System and Mental Health

Reproductive Systems

Respiratory System

The Senses

Urinary System

Word Building Example:

pantalgia
(pant-algia)

Pain involving the entire body.

---

papule

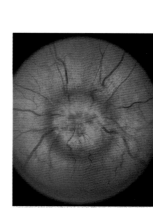

Word Building Example:

papulosis
(papul-osis)

The occurrence of numerous widespread papules.

---

relating to the wall
of any cavity;
somatic

Word Building Example:

parietal pleura
(pariet-al) pleura

The serous membrane that lines the different parts of the
wall of the pulmonary cavity.

Word Building Example:

pancreatitis
(pancreat-itis)

Inflammation of the pancreas.

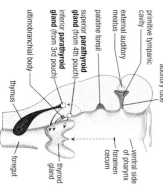

---

nipple-like;
optic disk

Word Building Example:

papilledema
(papill-edema)

Edema of the optic disc, often due to increased
intracranial pressure.

---

parathyroid

Word Building Example:

parathyroid gland
(parathyr-oid) gland

One of two small paired endocrine glands, superior and
inferior, usually found embedded in the connective tissue
capsule on the posterior surface of the thyroid gland.

auditory tube

primitive tympanic
cavity

external auditory
meatus

palatine tonsil

superior **parathyroid**
gland (from 4th pouch)

inferior **parathyroid**
gland (from 3rd pouch)

ultimobranchial body

thymus

foregut

thyroid
gland

cecum

foramen

ventral side
of pharynx

path/o, -pathy

General Terminology

Combining Form

ped/i, ped/o,
ped/a

General Terminology

Combining Form

Urinary System

perine/o

Combining Form

patell/o

Musculoskeletal System

Combining Form

Prefix

Combining Form

Suffix

pector/o

Musculoskeletal System

Combining Form

Blood and the Immune System

Cardiovascular System

Endocrine System

Gastrointestinal System

General Terminology

Integumentary System

pelv/i, pelv/o,
pelvi/o

Musculoskeletal System

Reproductive Systems

Combining Form

Musculoskeletal System

Nervous System and Mental Health

Reproductive Systems

Respiratory System

The Senses

Urinary System

disease

pathogenicity
(patho-gen-icity)

The condition or quality of being pathogenic, or the ability to cause disease.

---

knee cap

Word Building Example:

patella alta
(patell-a) alta

Term used to describe a somewhat more proximal position of the patella than anticipated when it is visualized on a lateral radiograph of the knee.

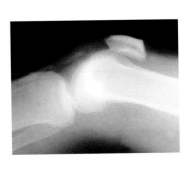

---

child;
foot, feet

Word Building Example:

pedatrophy
(peda-trophy)

A general weight loss and wasting, especially in young children, primarily due to prolonged dietary deficiency of protein and calories.

---

chest

Word Building Example:

pectoral
(pector-al)

Relating to the chest.

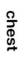
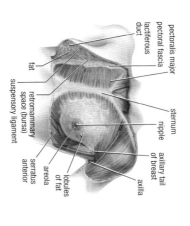

pectoralis major
pectoral fascia
lactiferous duct
fat
retromammary space (bursa)
suspensory ligament
sternum
nipple
axillary tail of breast
axilla
serratus anterior
areola
lobules of fat

---

perineum

Word Building Example:

perineocele
(perineo-cele)

---

pelvis

Word Building Example:

pelvicephalometry
(pelvi-cephalo-metry)

Measurement of the female pelvic diameters in relation to the fetal head.

Card 626

peritone/o

Gastrointestinal System

Combining Form

Card 628

petr/o

General Terminology

Combining Form

Card 630

phag/o

Gastrointestinal System

Combining Form

Card 625

perioste/o

Musculoskeletal System

Prefix
Combining Form
Suffix

Card 627

perone/o

Musculoskeletal System
Cardiovascular System

Combining Form

Blood and the Immune System
Cardiovascular System
Endocrine System
Gastrointestinal System
General Terminology
Integumentary System

Card 629

phac/o, phak/o

The Senses

Combining Form

Musculoskeletal System
Nervous System and Mental Health
Reproductive Systems
Respiratory System
The Senses
Urinary System

peritoneum

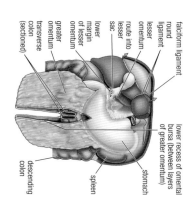

falciform ligament
round ligament
lesser omentum
lower margin of lesser sac
route into lesser sac
greater omentum
transverse colon (sectioned)
descending colon
spleen
stomach
lower recess of omental bursa (between layers of greater omentum)

peritonitis
(periton-itis)

Inflammation of the peritoneum.

---

stone, stone-like hardness

petromastoid
(petro-mast-oid)

Relating to the petrous and the squamous portions of the temporal bone.

---

eat or swallow

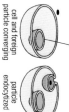
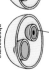

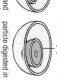

cell and foreign particle converging

lysosome

particle endocytized

phagosome and lysosome fused

phagosome approaching lysosome

secondary lysosome

phagosome

particle digested in secondary lysosome

phagocytosis
(phago-cyt-osis)

The process of ingestion and digestion by cells of solid substances.

---

periosteum

periosteum
(perioste-um)

The thick, fibrous membrane covering the entire surface of a bone except its articular cartilage.

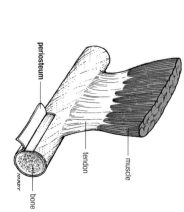

periosteum
tendon
muscle
bone

---

fibula

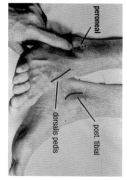

peroneal
dorsalis pedis
post. tibial

peroneal artery
(perone-al) artery

Origin, posterior tibial; distribution, courses deep to the flexor hallucis longus, supplying it and the soleus, tibialis posterior, fibularis muscles; inferior tibiofibular articulation, ankle joint, and lateral heel; anastomoses, anterior lateral malleolar, lateral tarsal, lateral plantar, dorsalis pedis.

---

lens-shaped, relating to a lens

phacocele
(phaco-cele)

Hernia of the lens of the eye through the sclera.

phaner/o

General Terminology

phall/i, phall/o

Reproductive Systems
Urinary System

Prefix
Combining Form
Suffix

pharyng/o

Combining Form

The Senses
Gastrointestinal System

pharmac/o

Combining Form

General Terminology

Blood and the Immune System
Cardiovascular System
Endocrine System
Gastrointestinal System
General Terminology
Integumentary System

phleb/o

Combining Form

Cardiovascular System

phe/o

Combining Form

General Terminology

Musculoskeletal System
Nervous System and Mental Health
Reproductive Systems
Respiratory System
The Senses
Urinary System

visible, obvious

penis

Word Building Example:

phanerosis
(phaner-osis)

The act or process of becoming visible.

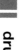

pharynx

Word Building Example:

phallodynia
(phallo-dynia)

Pain in the penis.

drugs

Word Building Example:

pharyngectomy
(pharyng-ectomy)

Resection of the pharynx.

Word Building Example:

pharmacomania
(pharmaco-mania)

Morbid impulse to take drugs.

vein

gray, dark-colored

Word Building Example:

phlebosclerosis
(phlebo-scler-osis)

Fibrous hardening of the walls of the veins.

Word Building Example:

pheochromocyte
(pheo-chromo-cyte)

A chromaffin cell of a sympathetic paraganglion, medulla of an adrenal gland, or a pheochromocytoma.

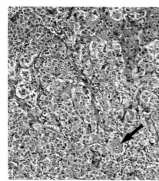

phor/o

General Terminology

phon/o

The Senses

Prefix

Combining Form

Suffix

Combining Form

phren/o, phrenic/o

General Terminology

Nervous System & Mental Health

Combining Form

phot/o

The Senses

Combining Form

Blood and the Immune System

Cardiovascular System

Endocrine System

Gastrointestinal System

General Terminology

Integumentary System

Combining Form

physi/o

General Terminology

Combining Form

phys/o

Endocrine System

Combining Form

Musculoskeletal System

Nervous System and Mental Health

Reproductive Systems

Respiratory System

The Senses

Urinary System

Combining Form

carrying, bearing;
a carrier, a bearer

Word Building Example:

phoria
(phor-ia)

The relative directions assumed by the eyes during binocular fixation of a given object in the absence of an adequate fusion stimulus.

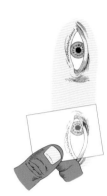

---

sound, speech

Word Building Example:

phonation
(phon-ation)

The production of sounds by vibration of the vocal folds.

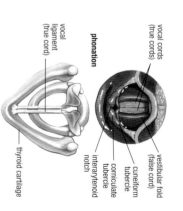

phonation

vocal cords
(true cords)

vocal
ligament
(true cord)

vestibular fold
(false cord)

cuneiform
tubercle

corniculate
tubercle

interarytenoid
notch

thyroid cartilage

---

diaphragm;
the mind

Word Building Example:

phrenocardia
(phreno-card-ia)

Precordial pain and dyspnea of psychogenic origin, often a symptom of anxiety neurosis.

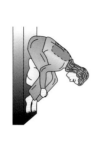

---

physical, physiological;
natural, relating to physics

Word Building Example:

physiotherapy
(physio-therapy)

Treatment of pain, disease, or injury by physical means

---

light

Word Building Example:

photodermatitis
(photo-dermat-itis)

Dermatitis caused or elicited by exposure to sunlight; may be phototoxic or photoallergic, and can also result from topical application, ingestion, inhalation, or injection of mediating phototoxic or photoallergic material.

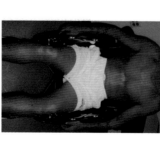

---

tendency to swell
or inflate

Word Building Example:

physometra
(physo-metr-a)

Distention of the uterine cavity with air or gas.

pil/o

Integumentary System

phyt/o

Integumentary System

Prefix
Combining Form
Suffix

---

pituitar/o

Combining Form

Endocrine System

pimel/o

Combining Form

General Terminology

Blood and the Immune System
Cardiovascular System
Endocrine System
Gastrointestinal System
General Terminology
Integumentary System

---

plant/o

Combining Form

Musculoskeletal System

plan/i, plan/o

Combining Form

General Terminology

Musculoskeletal System
Nervous System and Mental Health
Reproductive Systems
Respiratory System
The Senses
Urinary System

Word Building Example:

pilocystic

(pilo-cyst-ic)

Denoting a dermoid cyst containing hair.

Word Building Example:

phytodermatitis

(phyto-dermat-itis)

Dermatitis caused by mechanical and chemical injury, allergy, or photosensitization at skin sites previously exposed to plants.

**pituitary gland
(hypophysis)**

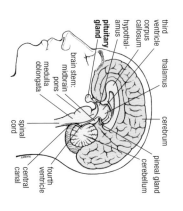

third ventricle
corpus callosum
hypothal-amus
pituitary gland

thalamus

brain stem:
midbrain
pons
medulla oblongata

spinal cord

cerebrum

pineal gland
cerebellum

central canal

fourth ventricle

fat, fatty

Word Building Example:

pituitary gland

(pituitar-y) gland

An unpaired compound gland suspended from the base of the hypothalamus by a short extension of the infundibulum, the infundibular or pituitary stalk.

Word Building Example:

pimelorthopnea

(pimel-ortho-pnea)

Orthopnea, difficulty breathing in any but the erect posture, due to obesity.

sole of foot

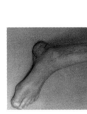

a plane, flat, level

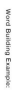

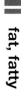

Word Building Example:

planimeter

(plani-meter)

An instrument formed of jointed levers with a recording index, used for measuring the area of any surface, by tracing its boundaries.

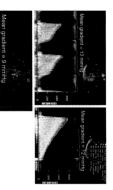

Mean gradient = 9 mmHg

Mean gradient = 13 mmHg

Mean gradient = 12 mmHg

Word Building Example:

plantigrade

(planti-grade)

Walking with the entire sole and heel of the foot on the ground, as humans and bears do.

ple/o

General Terminology

plasm/a, plasm/o, plasmat/o

General Terminology

Prefix
Combining Form
Suffix

pleur/a, pleur/o

Combining Form

Respiratory System
Cardiovascular System

pless/i

General Terminology

Combining Form

Blood and the Immune System
Cardiovascular System
Endocrine System
Gastrointestinal System
General Terminology
Integumentary System

pod/o

Combining Form

Musculoskeletal System

pneum/a, pneum/o, pneumat/o, pneumon/o

Respiratory System

Combining Form

Musculoskeletal System
Nervous System and Mental Health
Reproductive Systems
Respiratory System
The Senses
Urinary System

more

plasma

formative, organized; plasma

pleocytosis
(pleo-cyt-osis)

Presence of more cells than normal, often denoting leukocytosis and especially lymphocytosis or round cell infiltration.

plasmodium
(plasmo-dium)

Protoplasmic mass with several nuclei, due to multiplication of the nucleus with cell division.

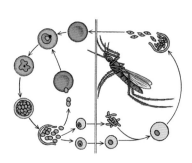

rib, side, pleura

striking, percussion

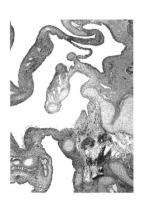

pleuropulmonary blastoma
(pleuro-pulmon-ary) blastoma

Blastoma of the pleura and lungs.

plessimeter
(plessi-meter)

Historic term for an oblong flexible plate used in mediate percussion by being placed against the surface and struck with the plessor.

foot

presence of air or gas; lung

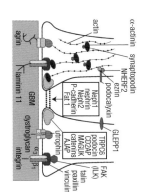

podocyte
(podo-cyte)

The modified epithelial cell of the visceral layer of glomerular capsule in the renal corpuscle, attached to the outer surface of the glomerular capillary basement membrane by cytoplasmic foot processes (pedicels).

pneumonitis
(pneumon-itis)

Inflammation of the lungs.

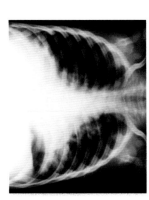

pon/o

General Terminology

poikil/o

Combining Form

Blood and the Immune System

Prefix

Combining Form

Suffix

poster/o

Combining Form

General Terminology

por/o

Combining Form

General Terminology

Integumentary System

Blood and the Immune System

Cardiovascular System

Endocrine System

Gastrointestinal System

General Terminology

Integumentary System

press/o

Combining Form

General Terminology

presby/o

Combining Form

General Terminology

The Senses

Musculoskeletal System

Nervous System and Mental Health

Reproductive Systems

Respiratory System

The Senses

Urinary System

bodily exertion, fatigue, overwork, pain

Word Building Example:
ponopalmosis
(pono-palm-osis)

Rarely used term for a condition of irritable heart in which palpitation is excited by slight exertion.

---

posterior, at the back of

Word Building Example:
posteroanterior
(postero-anteri-or)

A term denoting the direction of view or progression, from posterior to anterior, through a part.

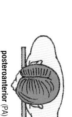
posteroanterior (PA)

---

pressure

Word Building Example:
compression
(com-press-ion)

The exertion of pressure on a body in such a way as to tend to increase its density

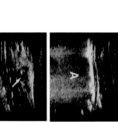
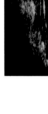

Technique of graded **compression**

---

irregular, varied

Word Building Example:
poikilocyte
(poikilo-cyte)

A red blood cell of irregular shape.

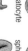
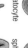

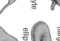

echinocyte
drepanocyte (holly leaf)
keratocyte (helmet cell)
dacryocyte (teardrop)
stomatocyte
schistocyte
acanthocyte
drepanocyte (sickle cell)
spherocyte
codocyte (target cell)
elliptocyte
knizocyte

---

a pore, a duct, an opening; going through, a passing through

Word Building Example:
porokeratosis
(poro-kerat-osis)

A rare dermatosis in which there is a thickening of the stratum corneum with an anular keratotic rim or cornoid lamella surrounding progressive centrifugal atrophy.

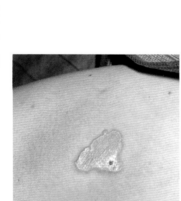

---

old age

Word Building Example:
presbyopia
(presby-opia)

The physiologic loss of accommodation in the eyes in advancing age, said to begin when the near point has receded beyond 22 cm (9 inches).

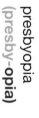
presbyopia
focal point of light rays: behind the retina

prosop/o

Musculoskeletal System

proct/o

Urinary System

| Prefix |
| Combining Form |
| Suffix |

prot/o, prote/o

Combining Form

General Terminology

prostat/o

Combining Form

Urinary System

| Blood and the Immune System |
| Cardiovascular System |
| Endocrine System |
| Gastrointestinal System |
| General Terminology |
| Integumentary System |

psych/o

Combining Form

Nervous System & Mental Health

prox/i, proxim/o

Combining Form

General Terminology

| Musculoskeletal System |
| Nervous System and Mental Health |
| Reproductive Systems |
| Respiratory System |
| The Senses |
| Urinary System |

the face

prosopalgia
(prosop-algia)

Facial pain.

---

protein;
first in a series;
highest in rank

proteolysis
(proteo-lysis)

Decomposition of protein.

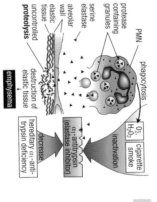

---

the mind, mental, psychologic

psychobiology
(psycho-bio-logy)

The study of the interrelationships of biology and
psychology in cognitive functioning, including intellectual,

---

anus; more frequently, rectum

proctococcypexy
(procto-coccy-pexy)

Suture of a prolapsing rectum to the tissues anterior
to the coccyx.

---

prostate gland

prostanoid
(prosta-noid)

Denoting having properties of prostaglandins.

---

proximal, nearest, next to

proximoataxia
(proximo-a-tax-ia)

Ataxia or lack of muscular coordination in the proximal
portions of the extremities (i.e., arms and thighs).

Card 668

pub/o

Reproductive Systems
Urinary System

Card 667

pter/o, pteryg/o

The Senses

Prefix
Combining Form
Suffix

Card 670

pupill/o

Combining Form

The Senses

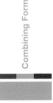

Card 669

pulm/o, pulmon/o

Combining Form

Respiratory System

Blood and the Immune System
Cardiovascular System
Endocrine System
Gastrointestinal System
General Terminology
Integumentary System

Card 672

pyel/o

Combining Form

Card 671

py/o

Combining Form

Urinary System

General Terminology

Musculoskeletal System
Nervous System and Mental Health
Reproductive Systems
Respiratory System
The Senses
Urinary System

pubis

Word Building Example:

**pubofemoral ligament
(pubo-femor-al) ligament**

A thickened part of the capsule of the hip joint that extends from the superior ramus of the pubis to the intertrochanteric line of the femur.

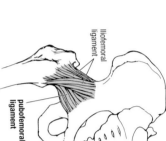

wing or feather; wing-shaped, usually relating to the pterygoid process

Word Building Example:

**pterygium
(pteryg-ium)**

A triangular patch of hypertrophied bulbar subconjunctival tissue.

---

pupils

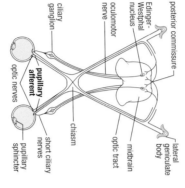

posterior commissure
Edinger-Westphal nucleus
oculomotor nerve
ciliary ganglion
optic nerves
pupillary afferent
short ciliary nerves
pupillary sphincter
chiasm
optic tract
midbrain
lateral geniculate body

lungs

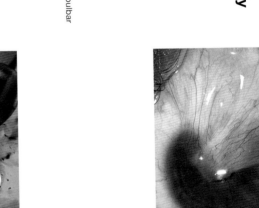

Word Building Example:

**pulmonic valve
(pulmon-ic) valve**

The valve at the entrance to the pulmonary trunk from the right ventricle.

Word Building Example:

**pupillary afferent fibers
(pupill-ary) afferent fibers**

Fibers that convey impulses from the pupil to a ganglion or to a nerve center in the brain or spinal cord.

pelvis, usually the renal pelvis

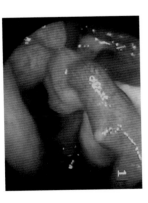

Word Building Example:

**pyelography
(pyelo-graphy)**

Radiologic study of the kidney, ureters, and usually the

suppuration, accumulation of pus

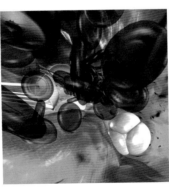

Word Building Example:

**pyosalpinx
(pyo-salpinx)**

Distention of a uterine (fallopian) tube with pus.

pyr/o, pyret/o

General Terminology

pylor/o

Gastrointestinal System

Prefix
Combining Form
Suffix

---

radi/o

Combining Form

General Terminology

rachi/o

Musculoskeletal System
Nervous System & Mental Health

Combining Form

Blood and the Immune System
Cardiovascular System
Endocrine System
Gastrointestinal System
General Terminology
Integumentary System

---

rect/o

Combining Form

radicul/o

Combining Form

Urinary System

Musculoskeletal System
Nervous System & Mental Health

Combining Form

Musculoskeletal System
Nervous System and Mental Health
Reproductive Systems
Respiratory System
The Senses
Urinary System

Word Building Example:

pyrosis
(pyr-osis)

A substernal pain or burning sensation, usually associated with regurgitation of acid and peptic gastric juice into the esophagus.

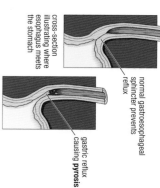

normal gastroesophageal sphincter prevents reflux

cross-section illustrating where esophagus meets the stomach

gastric reflux causing **pyrosis**

Word Building Example:

pyloroplasty
(pyloro-plasty)

Widening of the pyloric canal and any adjacent duodenal stricture by means of a longitudinal incision closed transversely.

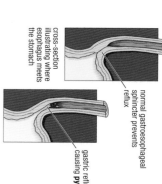

radiation, gamma
or x-ray;
radius

spine

Word Building Example:

radioimmunoassay
(radio-immuno-assay)

Any method for detecting or quantitating antigens or antibodies using radiolabeled reactants.

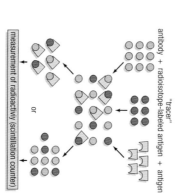

antibody + radioisotope-labeled antigen + antigen

"tracer"

or

measurement of radioactivity (scintillation counter)

rectum

root of spinal nerve

Word Building Example:

rachiocentesis
(rachio-centesis)

A puncture into the subarachnoid space of the lumbar region to obtain spinal fluid for diagnostic or therapeutic purposes.

Word Building Example:

rectoabdominal
(recto-abdomin-al)

Relating to the rectum and the abdomen.

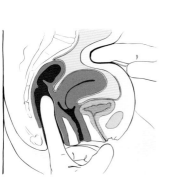

Rectoabdominal examination

Word Building Example:

radiculopathy
(radiculo-pathy)

Disorder of the spinal nerve roots.

reticul/o

General Terminology

ren/o, ren/i

Urinary System

Prefix

Combining Form

Suffix

rhabd/o

Combining Form

Musculoskeletal System

retin/o

Combining Form

The Senses

Blood and the Immune System

Cardiovascular System

Endocrine System

Gastrointestinal System

General Terminology

Integumentary System

rhin/o

Combining Form

The Senses

rheumat/o

Combining Form

Musculoskeletal System

Musculoskeletal System

Nervous System and Mental Health

Reproductive Systems

Respiratory System

The Senses

Urinary System

network

reticulocytosis
(reticulo-cyt-osis)

Word Building Example:

An increase in the number of circulating reticulocytes above the normal, which is less than 1.

rod, rod-shaped

rhabdomyosarcoma
(rhabdo-myo-sarc-oma)

Word Building Example:

A malignant neoplasm derived from skeletal (striated) muscle, occurring in children or, less commonly, in adults; classified as embryonal alveolar (composed of loose aggregates of small round cells) or pleomorphic (containing rhabdomyoblasts).

nose

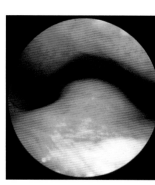

rhinoscopic view
(rhino-scop-ic) view

Word Building Example:

Endoscopic inspection of the nasal cavity.

---

kidney

renogram
(reno-gram)

Word Building Example:

The assessment of renal function by external radiation detectors after the administration of a radiopharmaceutical agent that is filtered and excreted by the kidney.

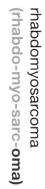

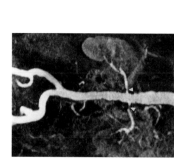

retina

retinoblastoma
(retino-blast-oma)

Word Building Example:

Malignant ocular neoplasm of childhood, usually occurring before the third year of life, composed of primitive retinal small round cells with deeply staining nuclei and of elongated cells forming rosettes.

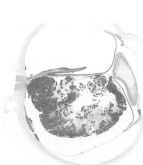

watery fluid

rheumatology
(rheumato-logy)

Word Building Example:

The medical specialty concerned with the study, diagnosis, and treatment of rheumatic conditions.

rhytid/o

General Terminology

Combining Form

sacchar/o

General Terminology

Combining Form

Reproductive Systems

The Senses

salping/o

Combining Form

rhiz/o

Musculoskeletal System

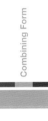

Prefix

Combining Form

Suffix

Combining Form

General Terminology

rubr/i, rubr/o

Combining Form

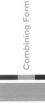

Blood and the Immune System

Cardiovascular System

Endocrine System

Gastrointestinal System

General Terminology

Integumentary System

sacr/o

Musculoskeletal System

Combining Form

Musculoskeletal System

Nervous System and Mental Health

Reproductive Systems

Respiratory System

The Senses

Urinary System

wrinkle

Word Building Example:

rhytidectomy
(rhytid-ectomy)

Elimination of wrinkles from, or reshaping of, the face by excising any excess skin and tightening the remainder.

---

sugar

Word Building Example:

saccharolytic
(saccharo-lytic)

Capable of hydrolyzing or otherwise breaking down a sugar molecule.

---

uterine tube;
eustachian tube

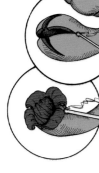
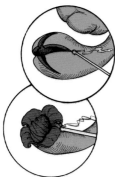

Word Building Example:

salpingostomy
(salpingo-stomy)

Establishment of an artificial opening in a uterine tube primarily as surgical treatment for an ectopic pregnancy.

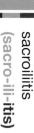

root

incision

area of
sensory
loss

clip

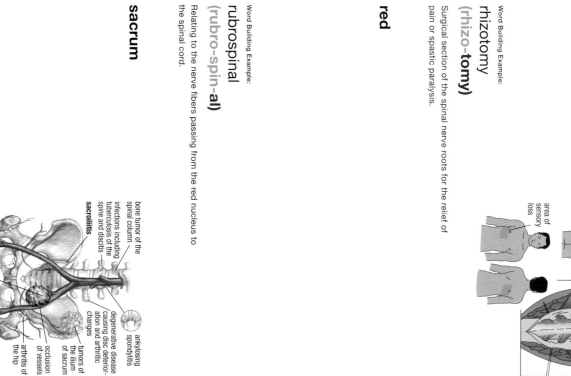

Word Building Example:

rhizotomy
(rhizo-tomy)

Surgical section of the spinal nerve roots for the relief of pain or spastic paralysis.

---

red

Word Building Example:

rubrospinal
(rubro-spin-al)

Relating to the nerve fibers passing from the red nucleus to the spinal cord.

---

sacrum

Word Building Example:

sacroiliitis
(sacro-ili-itis)

Inflammation of the sacroiliac joint.

bone tumor of the
spinal column

infections including
tuberculosis of the
spine and discitis

sacroiliitis

ankylosing
spondylitis

degenerative disease
causing disc deterior-
ation and arthritic
changes

tumors of
the ilium
of sacrum

occlusion
of vessels

arthritis of
the hip

infrapelvic mass
(abscess, tumor)

sarc/o

General Terminology

Prefix

Combining Form

Suffix

scaph/o

Musculoskeletal System

Combining Form

---

scapul/o

Musculoskeletal System

Blood and the Immune System

Cardiovascular System

Endocrine System

Gastrointestinal System

General Terminology

Integumentary System

Combining Form

scat/o

Urinary System

Combining Form

---

schist/o

General Terminology

Musculoskeletal System

Nervous System and Mental Health

Reproductive Systems

Respiratory System

The Senses

Urinary System

Combining Form

schiz/o, schist/o

General Terminology

Nervous System & Mental Health

Combining Form

scaphoid, boat-shaped, hollowed

scaphoid
(scaph-oid)

Boat-shaped; hollowed.

feces

scatoscopy
(scato-scopy)

Examination of the feces for purposes of diagnosis.

split, cleft, division

schistothorax
(schisto-thorax)

Congenital cleft of the chest wall

muscular substance;
a resemblance to flesh

Carpometacarpal joints, articular surfaces.
Anterior view of the articular surfaces of
the carpometacarpal joints (HH, hook of
hamate; H, hamate; C, Capitate; Td, trapezoid;
Tz, trapezium; S, **scaphoid**; L, lunate; Tq,
triquetrum; P, pisiform)

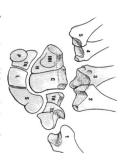

sarcoidosis
(sarc-oid-osis)

A systemic granulomatous disease of unknown cause,
especially involving the lungs with resulting fibrosis, but
also involving lymph nodes, skin, liver, spleen, eyes,
phalangeal bones, and parotid glands.

scapula (shoulder blade)

scapulohumeral
(scapulo-humer-al)

Relating to both scapula and humerus.

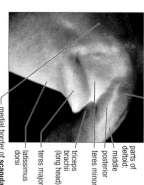

trapezius (superior fibers)
parts of
deltoid:
middle
posterior
teres minor
triceps
brachii
(long head)
teres major
latissimus
dorsi
medial border of **scapula**

cleft, division

schistocyte
(schisto-cyte)

A poikilocyte that owes its abnormal shape to
fragmentation as the cell flows through damaged small
vessels.

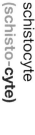

scler/o

General Terminology
The Senses

scirrh/o

General Terminology

Prefix

Combining Form

Suffix

scot/o

Combining Form

The Senses

scoli/o

Combining Form

Musculoskeletal System

Blood and the Immune System

Cardiovascular System

Endocrine System

Gastrointestinal System

General Terminology

Integumentary System

semin/i

Combining Form

Reproductive Systems

seb/i, seb/o

Combining Form

Integumentary System

Musculoskeletal System

Nervous System and Mental Health

Reproductive Systems

Respiratory System

The Senses

Urinary System

Word Building Example:

scleroderma
(sclero-derma)

Dermal thickening and induration due to new collagen formation, with atrophy of pilosebaceous follicles.

---

darkness

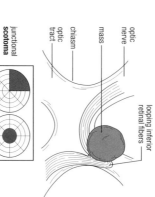

optic nerve

chiasm

optic tract

mass

looping inferior retinal fibers

junctional **scotoma**

Word Building Example:

scotoma
(scoto-oma)

1. An isolated area of varying size and shape, within the visual field, in which vision is absent or depressed. 2. A blind spot in psychological awareness.

---

semen

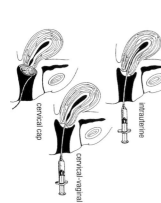

cervical cap

cervical-vaginal

intrauterine

Word Building Example:

insemination
(in-semin-ation)

Deposit of seminal fluid within the vagina, normally during coitus.

---

hard

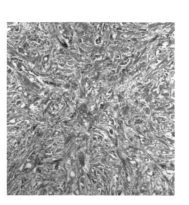

Word Building Example:

scirrhous
(scirrh-ous)

Hard; relating to a scirrhus, a hard tumor.

---

crooked

Word Building Example:

scoliometer
(scolio-meter)

An instrument for measuring curves, especially those in lateral curvature of the spine.

---

sebum, sebaceous
(secretion of the sebaceous glands), tallow

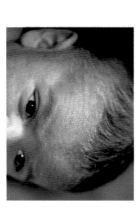

Word Building Example:

seborrhea
(sebo-rrhea)

Overactivity of the sebaceous glands, resulting in an excessive amount of sebum.

sept/o, sept/i, septic/o

Respiratory System

sider/o

General Terminology

Combining Form

silic/o, silic/i

General Terminology

Combining Form

sens/o, sens/i

The Senses

Prefix

Combining Form

Suffix

sial/o

Combining Form

Gastrointestinal System

The Senses

Blood and the Immune System

Cardiovascular System

Endocrine System

Gastrointestinal System

General Terminology

Integumentary System

sigmoid/o

Combining Form

Gastrointestinal System

Musculoskeletal System

Nervous System and Mental Health

Reproductive Systems

Respiratory System

The Senses

Urinary System

Word Building Example:

septicemia
(septic-emia)

Systemic disease caused by the spread of microorganisms and their toxins through circulating blood; formerly called "blood poisoning."

Word Building Example:

sensigenous
(sensi-gen-ous)

Giving rise to sensation.

iron

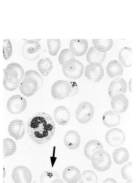

saliva, salivary glands

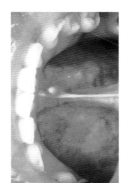

Word Building Example:

siderosis
(sider-osis)

1. Pneumoconiosis due to the presence of iron dust. 2. Discoloration of any part by deposition of a pigment containing iron; usually called hemosiderosis. 3. An excess of iron in the circulating blood. 4. Degeneration of the retina, lens, and uvea as a result of the deposition of intraocular iron.

Word Building Example:

sialolithiasis
(sialo-lith-iasis)

The formation or presence of a salivary calculus.

silica or silicon

sigmoid, usually the sigmoid colon

Word Building Example:

silicosis
(silic-osis)

A form of pneumoconiosis resulting from occupational exposure to and inhalation of silica dust over a period of years.

Word Building Example:

sigmoidoscope
(sigmoido-scope)

An endoscope for viewing the cavity of the sigmoid colon.

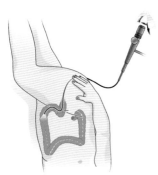

sinistr/o

General Terminology

sin/o

Respiratory System

Prefix

Combining Form

Suffix

soci/o

Combining Form

Nervous System & Mental Health

sinus/o

Respiratory System

Combining Form

Blood and the Immune System

Cardiovascular System

Endocrine System

Gastrointestinal System

General Terminology

Integumentary System

somn/i, somn/o

Combining Form

som/o, somat/o

General Terminology

Combining Form

General Terminology

Nervous System & Mental Health

Musculoskeletal System

Nervous System and Mental Health

Reproductive Systems

Respiratory System

The Senses

Urinary System

Word Building Example:

sinistrocardia
(sinistro-card-ia)

Displacement of the heart beyond the normal position on the left side.

---

social, society

Word Building Example:

socioacusis
(socio-acusis)

The hearing loss produced by exposure to nonoccupational noise such as small arms fire in hunting and target practice.

---

sleep

Word Building Example:

insomnia
(in-somn-ia)

Inability to sleep, in the absence of external impediments during the period when sleep should normally occur; may vary in degree from restlessness or disturbed slumber to a curtailment of the normal length of sleep to absolute wakefulness.

Word Building Example:

sinovaginal
(sino-vagin-al)

Relating to that part of the vagina derived from the urogenital sinus.

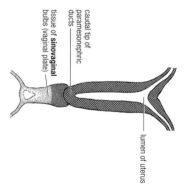

caudal tip of paramesonephric ducts

tissue of **sinovaginal** bulbs (vaginal plate)

lumen of uterus

---

hollow (cavity)

Word Building Example:

sinusitis
(sinus-itis)

Inflammation of the mucous membrane of any sinus, especially the paranasal.

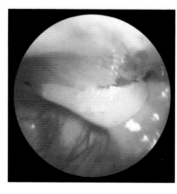

---

body, bodily

Word Building Example:

somatotype
(somato-type)

1. The constitutional or body type of a person. 2. The particular constitutional or body type associated with a particular personality type.

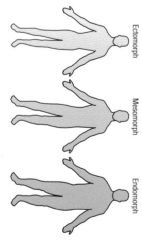

Ectomorph

Mesomorph

Endomorph

son/o

General Terminology

Prefix

Combining Form

Suffix

Combining Form

sperm/a, sperm/o, spermat/o, sperm/i

Reproductive Systems

Combining Form

sphen/o

Musculoskeletal System

Blood and the Immune System

Cardiovascular System

Endocrine System

Gastrointestinal System

General Terminology

Integumentary System

Combining Form

sphygm/o

General Terminology

Combining Form

spin/o

Musculoskeletal System

Nervous System & Mental Health

Musculoskeletal System

Nervous System and Mental Health

Reproductive Systems

Respiratory System

The Senses

Urinary System

Combining Form

spir/o

General Terminology

Respiratory System

Combining Form

semen, spermatozoa

Word Building Example:

spermatogenesis
(spermato-genesis)

The entire process by which spermatogonial stem cells divide and differentiate into sperms.

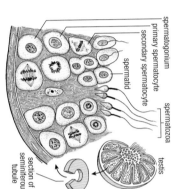

spermatogonium
primary spermatocyte
secondary spermatocyte
spermatid
spermatozoa
testis
section of seminiferous tubule

pulse

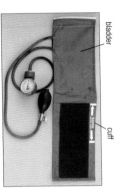

bladder

cuff

sound

Word Building Example:

sonography
(sono-graphy)

The location, measurement, or delineation of deep structures by measuring the reflection or transmission of high-frequency or ultrasonic waves.

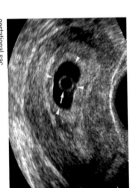

gestational sac

Word Building Example:

sphygmomanometer
(sphygmo-mano-meter)

An instrument to measure arterial blood pressure indirectly, with an inflatable cuff, inflating bulb, and a gauge to show blood pressure.

coil, coil-shaped; breathing

Word Building Example:

spirometry
(spiro-metry)

Making pulmonary measurements with a spirometer, a device used for measuring flows and volumes, inspired and

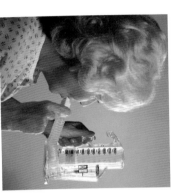

Word Building Example:

sphenoiditis
(sphen-oid-itis)

Inflammation of the sphenoid sinus.

the spine; spinous

Word Building Example:

spinomuscular
(spino-muscul-ar)

Relating to the spinal cord and the muscles supplied by the spinal nerves.

wedge, wedge-shaped; the sphenoid bone

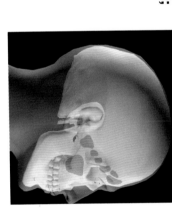

splen/o

Gastrointestinal System

Combining Form

General Terminology

spongi/o

Combining Form

General Terminology

squam/o

Combining Form

splanchn/i,
splanchn/o

Gastrointestinal System

Combining Form

Prefix

Combining Form

Suffix

spondyl/o

Musculoskeletal System

Nervous System & Mental Health

Combining Form

Blood and the Immune System

Cardiovascular System

Endocrine System

Gastrointestinal System

General Terminology

Integumentary System

spor/i, spor/o

General Terminology

Reproductive Systems

Combining Form

Musculoskeletal System

Nervous System and Mental Health

Reproductive Systems

Respiratory System

The Senses

Urinary System

splenomegaly
(spleno-megaly)

Enlargement of the spleen.

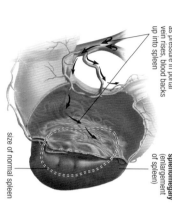

as pressure in portal vein rises, blood backs up into spleen

splenomegaly (enlargement of spleen)

size of normal spleen

splanchnocranium
(splanchno-crani-um)

That part of the cranium derived from the embryonic pharyngeal arches; comprises the facial bones of the facial skeleton (under bone) and is distinct from that part of the cranium that forms the neurocranium (braincase).

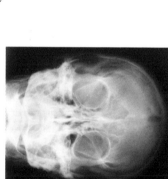

Word Building Example:

spongiosis
(spongi-osis)

1. Inflammatory intercellular edema of the epidermis. 2. In neurology, vacuolation of cortical grey matter seen in some encephalopathies.

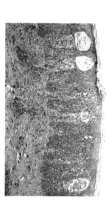

---

sponge, sponge-like, spongy

Word Building Example:

squamous cell carcinoma
(squamo-us) cell carcinoma

A malignant neoplasm derived from stratified squamous epithelium, but that may also occur in sites such as bronchial mucosa where glandular or columnar epithelium is normally present.

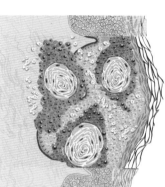

---

squama, squamous

Word Building Example:

spondylolysis
(spondylo-lysis)

Degeneration or deficient development of the articulating part of a vertebra.

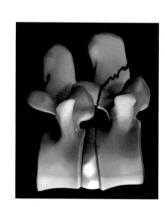

---

vertebrae

Word Building Example:

sporoblast
(sporo-blast)

An early stage in the development of a sporocyst before differentiation of the sporozoites.

---

seed, spore

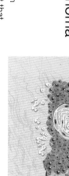

staphyl/o

General Terminology

staped/o, stapedi/o

The Senses

Prefix

Combining Form

Suffix

sten/o

Combining Form

General Terminology

steat/o

Combining Form

Gastrointestinal System

Integumentary System

Blood and the Immune System

Cardiovascular System

Endocrine System

Gastrointestinal System

General Terminology

Integumentary System

stern/o

Combining Form

Musculoskeletal System

Cardiovascular System

stere/o

Combining Form

General Terminology

Musculoskeletal System

Nervous System and Mental Health

Reproductive Systems

Respiratory System

The Senses

Urinary System

grapelike cluster, staphylococcus

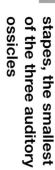

Word Building Example:

staphylococcal folliculitis
(staphylo-cocc-al)

An inflammation of a hair follicle, caused by any organism of the genus *Staphylococcus*.

---

narrowness, constriction

Word Building Example:

stenothorax
(steno-thorax)

A narrow, contracted chest.

---

the sternum, sternal

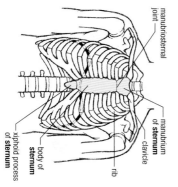
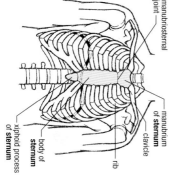

manubriosternal joint
manubrium of **sternum**
clavicle
body of **sternum**
rib
xiphoid process of **sternum**

Word Building Example:

sternum
(stern-um)

A long, flat bone, articulating with the cartilages of the first seven ribs and with the clavicle, that forms the middle part of the anterior wall of the thorax.

---

stapes, the smallest of the three auditory ossicles

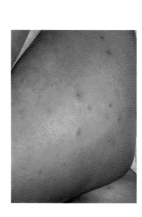

Word Building Example:

stapedius
(stapedi-us)

One of the muscles of the auditory ossicles.

tensor tympani muscle
stapedius muscle
tympanic membrane
round window
ossicles
cochlea
oval window

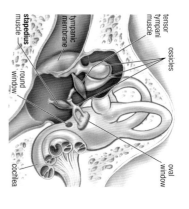

---

fat

Word Building Example:

steatonecrosis
(steato-necr-osis)

The death of adipose tissue, characterized by the formation of small (1–4 mm), dull, chalky, gray or white foci; these represent small quantities of calcium soaps formed in the affected tissue when fat is hydrolyzed into glycerol and fatty acids.

fibroadenoma
glandular tissue: gland lobules
intraductal papilloma
fat necrosis
glandular tissue: ampulla
glandular tissue: lactiferous duct
nipple

---

a solid condition or state denoting three-dimensionality

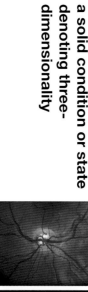
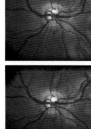

Word Building Example:

stereoscopic
(stereo-scop-ic)

Relating to a stereoscope, or giving the appearance of three dimensions.

Card 734

sthen/o

General Terminology

Card 733

steth/o

General Terminology

Prefix
Combining Form
Suffix

Card 736

styl/o

Combining Form

Musculoskeletal System

Card 735

stomat/o

Combining Form

Gastrointestinal System
The Senses

Blood and the Immune System
Cardiovascular System
Endocrine System
Gastrointestinal System
General Terminology
Integumentary System

Card 738

sympath/o, sympathet/o

Combining Form

Nervous System & Mental Health

Card 737

sudor/o

Combining Form

General Terminology

Musculoskeletal System
Nervous System and Mental Health
Reproductive Systems
Respiratory System
The Senses
Urinary System

strength

Word Building Example:

myosthenometer
(myo-stheno-meter)

An instrument for measuring the power of muscle groups.

---

chest

Word Building Example:

stethoscope
(stetho-scope)

An instrument originally devised by Laennec for aid in hearing the respiratory and cardiac sounds in the chest, but now modified in various ways and used in auscultation of any vascular or other sounds anywhere in the body.

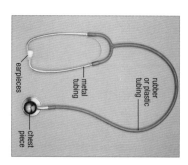

rubber or plastic tubing

metal tubing

earpieces

chest piece

---

styloid (specifically the styloid process of the temporal bone)

Word Building Example:

stylomandibular ligament
(stylo-mandibul-ar) ligament

A condensation of the deep cervical fascia extending from the tip of the styloid process of the temporal bone to the posterior border of the angle of the jaw.

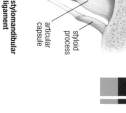

sphenomandibular ligament

mandibular foramen

styloid process

articular capsule

stylomandibular ligament

---

mouth

Word Building Example:

stomatocyte
(stomato-cyte)

A red blood cell that exhibits a slit or mouth-shaped pallor rather than a central one on air-dried smears.

---

the sympathetic part of the autonomic nervous system

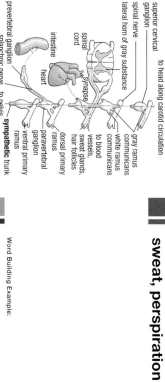

superior cervical ganglion

spinal nerve

lateral horn of gray substance

spinal cord

intestine

synapse

heart

prevertebral ganglion

splanchnic nerve

to head along carotid circulation

gray ramus communicans

white ramus communicans

to blood vessels, sweat glands, hair follicles

dorsal primary ramus

paravertebral ganglion

ventral primary ramus

to pelvis

sympathetic trunk

Word Building Example:

sympathetic
(sympathet-ic)

1. Relating to or exhibiting sympathy. 2. Denoting the sympathetic part of the autonomic nervous system.

---

sweat, perspiration

Word Building Example:

sudorrhea
(sudo-rrhea)

Excessive or profuse sweating.

synov/i

Musculoskeletal System

synapt/o

General Terminology

Nervous System & Mental Health

Prefix

Combining Form

Suffix

tax/o, taxi/o

Combining Form

General Terminology

tars/o

Combining Form

Musculoskeletal System

The Senses

Blood and the Immune System

Cardiovascular System

Endocrine System

Gastrointestinal System

General Terminology

Integumentary System

terat/o

Reproductive Systems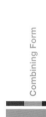

Combining Form

ten/o, tend/o, tendin/o

Combining Form

Musculoskeletal System

Musculoskeletal System

Nervous System and Mental Health

Reproductive Systems

Respiratory System

The Senses

Urinary System

synovial joint, synovial membrane

synovial fluid
(synovi-al) fluid

A clear thixotropic fluid, the main function of which is to serve as a lubricant in a joint, tendon sheath, or bursa.

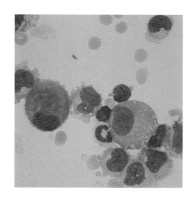

synapse

Word Building Example:

synaptophysin
(synapto-phys-in)

An integral membrane glycoprotein found in many types of active neurons; believed to form a hexamer that forms an ion channel and is involved in the uptake of neurotransmitters; synaptophysin is found in the membrane only after stimulation of the neurons.

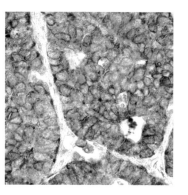

---

order, arrangement

Word Building Example:

ataxia
(a-tax-ia)

An inability to coordinate muscle activity, causing jerkiness, incoordination, and inefficiency of voluntary movement.

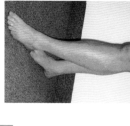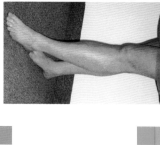

tarsus (as a division of the skeleton, the seven tarsal bones of the instep); tarsus (the fibrous plates giving solidity and form to the edges of the eyelids)

Word Building Example:

tarsorrhaphy
(tarso-rrhaphy)

Suturing together the eyelid margins, partially or completely, to shorten the palpebral fissure or to protect the cornea in keratitis.

---

malformed fetus

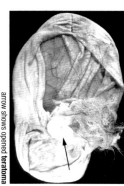

arrow shows opened **teratoma** revealing a solid knob from which hair projects

Word Building Example:

teratoma
(terat-oma)

A neoplasm composed of multiple tissues, including tissues not normally found in the organ in which it arises.

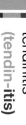

tendon

Word Building Example:

tendinitis
(tendin-itis)

Inflammation of a tendon.

Card 745

test/o

Reproductive Systems

Prefix
Combining Form
Suffix

Card 746

thalam/o

Combining Form

Nervous System & Mental Health

Card 747

thec/o

General Terminology

Blood and the Immune System
Cardiovascular System
Endocrine System
Gastrointestinal System
General Terminology
Integumentary System

Card 748

thel/o

Combining Form

General Terminology

Card 749

therm/o

General Terminology

Musculoskeletal System
Nervous System and Mental Health
Reproductive Systems
Respiratory System
The Senses
Urinary System

Card 750

thorac/o, thoracic/o

Combining Form

Musculoskeletal System
Cardiovascular System

thalamus

Word Building Example:
thalamotomy
(thalamo-tomy)

Destruction of a selected portion of the thalamus by stereotaxy for the relief of pain, involuntary movements, epilepsy, and, rarely, emotional disturbances.

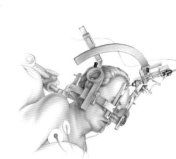

nipples

Word Building Example:
thelorrhagia
(thelo-rrhagia)

Bleeding form the nipple.

chest

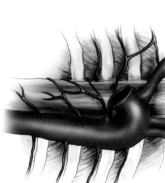

Word Building Example:
thoracic aorta
(thorac-ic) aorta

The part of the descending aorta that supplies structures as far down as the diaphragm.

testis, testicle

Word Building Example:
testicular
(test-icular)

Relating to the testes.

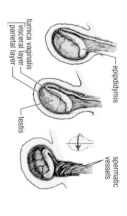

turnica vaginalis
visceral layer
parietal layer
epipdidymis
testis
spermatic vessels

sheath or capsule

Word Building Example:
ootheca
(oo-thec-a)

1. An egg case found in some lower animals. 2. Rarely used term for ovary.

heat, temperature

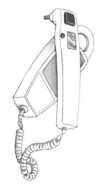

Word Building Example:
thermometer
(thermo-meter)

An instrument for indicating the temperature of any substance.

Card
752

thym/i, thym/o

Endocrine System

Nervous System & Mental Health

Card
754

tibi/o

Combining Form

Musculoskeletal System

Cardiovascular System

Card
756

tom/o

Combining Form

General Terminology

Combining Form

Card
751

thromb/o

Blood and the Immune System

Combining Form

Prefix

Combining Form

Suffix

Card
753

thyr/o, thyroid/o

Endocrine System

Combining Form

Blood and the Immune System

Cardiovascular System

Endocrine System

Gastrointestinal System

General Terminology

Integumentary System

Card
755

toc/o

Reproductive Systems

Combining Form

Musculoskeletal System

Nervous System and Mental Health

Reproductive Systems

Respiratory System

The Senses

Urinary System

thymus (a primary lymphoid organ);
mind, soul, emotions

Word Building Example:
thymitis
(thym-itis)

Inflammation of the thymus gland.

---

tibia, shinbone

---

to cut

Word Building Example:
tibiofibular
(tibio-fibul-ar)

Relating to both the tibia and fibula; denotes especially the joints and ligaments between the two bones.

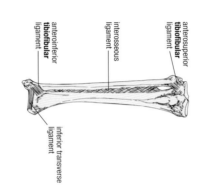

anterosuperior **tibiofibular** ligament

interosseous ligament

anteroinferior **tibiofibular** ligament

inferior transverse ligament

FRONT

Word Building Example:
tomogram
(tomo-gram)

A radiograph of a selected plane by means of reciprocal linear or curved motion of the X-ray tube and film cassette.

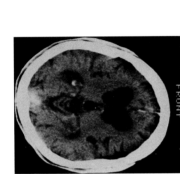

---

blood clot;
coagulation

Word Building Example:
thrombosis
(thromb-osis)

Clotting within a blood vessel that may cause infarction of tissues supplied by the vessel.

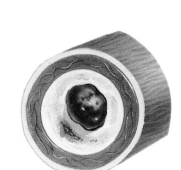

endothelium
smooth muscle
external elastic membrane

tunica intima
tunica media
tunica adventitia
thrombus
valve
internal elastic membrane

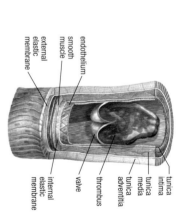

---

thyroid

Word Building Example:
thyroidectomy
(thyroid-ectomy)

Removal of the thyroid gland.

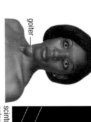

goiter

scintogram showing diffuse, enlarged thyroid gland

---

childbirth

Word Building Example:
tocolytic
(toco-lytic)

Denoting any pharmacologic agent used to arrest uterine contractions; often used to arrest premature labor contractions.

tonsill/o

The Senses

---

tox/i, tox/o, toxic/o

Combining Form

General Terminology

---

trich/o

Combining Form

Integumentary System

Combining Form

---

ton/o

General Terminology

Prefix

Combining Form

Suffix

---

top/o

Combining Form

General Terminology

Blood and the Immune System

Cardiovascular System

Endocrine System

Gastrointestinal System

General Terminology

Integumentary System

---

trache/o

Combining Form

Respiratory Systems

Combining Form

Musculoskeletal System

Nervous System and Mental Health

Reproductive Systems

Respiratory System

The Senses

Urinary System

tonsils

Word Building Example:
tonsillitis
(tonsill-itis)

Inflammation of a tonsil, especially of the palatine tonsil.

poison, toxin

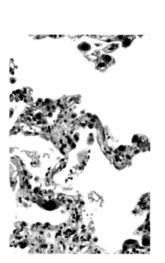

Word Building Example:
cytotoxic
(cyto-tox-ic)

Detrimental or destructive to cells.

hair, hair-like structure

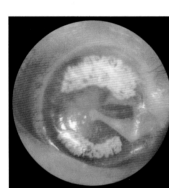
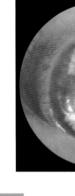

Word Building Example:
trichomoniasis
(tricho-mon-iasis)

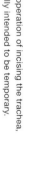

Disease caused by infection with a species of protozoon of the genus *Trichomonas* or related genera.

tone, tension, pressure

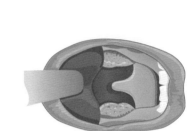

Word Building Example:
tonometer
(tono-meter)

An instrument for determining pressure or tension, especially an instrument for determining ocular tension.

place, topical

Word Building Example:
topognosis
(topo-gnosis)

Recognition of the location of a sensation.

trachea

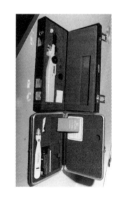

hyoid
thyroid cartilage
thyroid gland
tracheostomy
tube
inflation tube
expanding
ballon

preferred location
is between 2nd and
3rd tracheal rings
epiglottis
cricoid
trachea
1st tracheal
ring
esophagus

Word Building Example:
tracheostomy
(tracheo-stomy)

The operation of incising the trachea, usually intended to be temporary.

tub/o

Reproductive Systems

Combining Form

trigon/o

General Terminology

Combining Form

Prefix

Combining Form

Suffix

tympan/i,
tympan/o

Combining Form

The Senses

tuss/o

Combining Form

Respiratory System

Blood and the Immune System

Cardiovascular System

Endocrine System

Gastrointestinal System

General Terminology

Integumentary System

ul/e, ul/o

Combining Form

General Terminology
Gastrointestinal System

typhl/o

Combining Form

Gastrointestinal System
The Senses

Musculoskeletal System

Nervous System and Mental Health

Reproductive Systems

Respiratory System

The Senses

Urinary System

tubular, a tube

Word Building Example:
**tuboovarian abscess
(tubo-ovar-ian) abscess**

A large abscess involving a uterine tube and an adherent ovary, resulting from extension of purulent inflammation of the tube.

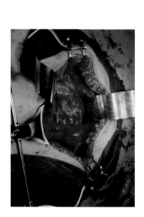

relating to a trigone, a triangular area

Word Building Example:
**trigonocephaly
(trigono-cephal-y)**

Malformation with a triangular cranial configuration, due in part to premature synostosis of the cranial bones with compression of the cerebral hemispheres.

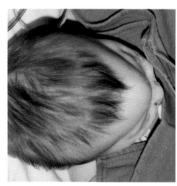

---

tympanum, tympanites

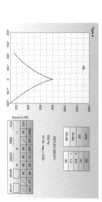

cough

Word Building Example:
**tympanogram
(tympano-gram)**

A visual depiction (e.g., a printout) of the relative compliance and impedance of the structures of the middle ear in response to pressure changes in the external ear canal.

Word Building Example:
**pertussis
(per-tuss-is)**

An acute infectious inflammation of the larynx, trachea, and bronchi caused by Bordetella pertussis; characterized by recurrent bouts of spasmodic coughing that continues until the breath is exhausted, then ending in a noisy inspiratory stridor (the "whoop") caused by laryngeal spasm.

---

scar, scarring; gums

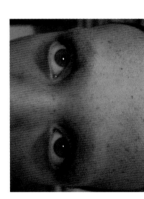

cecum; blindness

Word Building Example:
**ulerythema
(ul-eryth-ema)**

Scarring with erythema, redness due to capillary dilation.

Word Building Example:
**typhlomegaly
(typhlo-megaly)**

Old term for enlargement of the cecum.

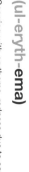

umbilic/o

General Terminology
Gastrointestinal System

Combining Form

Urinary System
Endocrine System

uln/o

Musculoskeletal System

Prefix
Combining Form
Suffix

ur/e, ur/o,
ure/a, ure/o

Combining Form

Urinary System

ungu/o

Integumentary System

Combining Form

Blood and the Immune System
Cardiovascular System
Endocrine System
Gastrointestinal System
General Terminology
Integumentary System

ureter/o

Combining Form

uran/o, uranisc/o

The Senses

Combining Form

Musculoskeletal System
Nervous System and Mental Health
Reproductive Systems
Respiratory System
The Senses
Urinary System

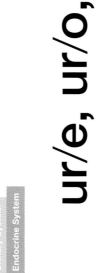
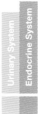
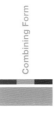
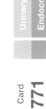

navel

umbilical cord
(umbilic-al) cord

Word Building Example:

The definitive connecting stalk between the embryo or fetus and the placenta.

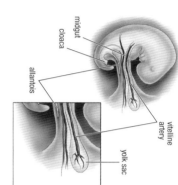

midgut
cloaca
allantois
vitelline
artery
yolk sac

relating to the ulna

ulnocarpal
(ulno-carp-al)

Word Building Example:

Relating to the ulna and the carpus, or to the ulnar side of the wrist.

A. Dorsal extrinsic ligaments of the wrist: dorsal intercarpal ligaments (DIC); dorsal radiotriquetral ligament (DRT); trapezium (Tm); trapezoid (Td); capitate (C); hamate (H); scaphoid (S); triquetrum (T). B. Volar extrinsic ligaments of the wrist: scaphotrapezial (ST); radioscaphocapitate (RSC); scaphocapitate (SC); long radiolunate (LRL); short radiolunate (SRL); **ulnocarpal** (UC); palmar lunatotriquetral (PLT); triquetral-capitate (TC); triquetral-hamate (TH); lunate (L); scaphoid (S); pisiform (P). C. Intrinsic ligaments of the wrist: scapholunate (SL); lunatotriquetral (LT); scaphotrapeziotrapezoidal (STT); lunatotriquetral (LT); scaphotrapeziotrapezoidal (STT); scaphocapitate (SC); triquetral capitate (TC); triquetral-hamate (TH); capitohamate (CH); capitotrapezoidal (CT); trapeziotrapezoidal (TT). C, capitate; S, scaphoid; L, lunate.

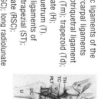

urea;
urine

The heart of a patient who died of **uremia** displays a shaggy, fibrinous exudate covering the visceral pericardium.

relating to a nail

ungulate
(ungu-late)

Word Building Example:

Having hooves.

uremia
(ur-emia)

Word Building Example:

1. An excess of urea and other nitrogenous waste in the blood. 2. The complex of symptoms due to severe persisting renal failure that can be relieved by dialysis.

ureter

the hard palate

uranostaphyloschisis
(urano-staphylo-schisis)

Word Building Example:

Cleft of the soft and hard palates.

ureterocele
(uretero-cele)

Word Building Example:

Saccular dilation of the terminal portion of the ureter that protrudes into the lumen of the urinary bladder, probably due to a congenital stenosis of the ureteral meatus.

urin/o

Urinary System

uve/o

Combining Form

The Senses

vag/o

Nervous System & Mental Health

Combining Form

urethr/o

Urinary System

Combining Form

Prefix

Combining Form

Suffix

uter/o

Reproductive Systems

Combining Form

Blood and the Immune System

Cardiovascular System

Endocrine System

Gastrointestinal System

General Terminology

Integumentary System

uvul/o

Gastrointestinal System

Combining Form

Musculoskeletal System

Nervous System and Mental Health

Reproductive Systems

Respiratory System

The Senses

Urinary System

urine

urinary tract
(urin-ary) tract

The passage from the pelvis of the kidney to the urinary meatus through the ureters, bladder, and urethra.

uvea (of eye)

uveoscleritis
(uveo-scler-itis)

Inflammation of the sclera involved by extension from the uvea.

vagus nerve

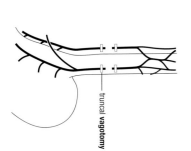

truncal **vagotomy**

vagotomy
(vago-tomy)

Division of the vagus nerve.

urethra

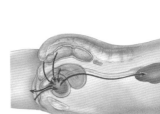

urethral groove
(urethr-al) groove

The groove on the ventral surface of the embryonic penis that ultimately is closed to form the spongy portion of the urethra.

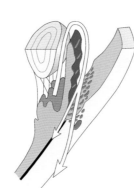

uterus

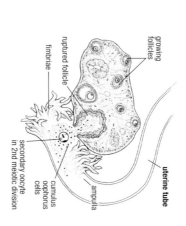

growing follicles

ruptured follicle

fimbriae

secondary oocyte in 2nd meiotic division

cumulus oophorus cells

ampulla

uterine tube

uterine tube
(uter-ine) tube

One of the tubes leading on either side from the upper or outer extremity of the ovary, which is largely enveloped by its expanded infundibulum, to the fundus of the uterus.

uvula

uvulotome
(uvulo-tome)

An instrument for cutting the uvula.

phallus

urethral groove

scrotal swellings

urethral fold

perineum

anal folds

penile urethra

solid epithelial cord

glandular part of urethra

urethral plate

urethral outlet

glans penis

line of fusion of urethral folds

line of fusion of scrotal swellings (scrotal septum)

lumen of penile urethra

perineum

anus

Card
781

vagin/o

Reproductive Systems

Prefix

Combining Form

Suffix

Card
782

valv/o, valvul/o

Cardiovascular System

Combining Form

Card
783

varic/o

Cardiovascular System

Blood and the Immune System

Cardiovascular System

Endocrine System

Gastrointestinal System

General Terminology

Integumentary System

Combining Form

Card
784

vas/o, vascul/o

Cardiovascular System

Combining Form

General Terminology

Card
785

ven/o, ven/i

Cardiovascular System

Musculoskeletal System

Nervous System and Mental Health

Reproductive Systems

Respiratory System

The Senses

Urinary System

Combining Form

Card
786

ventr/o

Combining Form

valve

valvuloplasty
(valvulo-plasty)

Surgical reconstruction of a deformed cardiac valve, for the relief of stenosis or incompetence.

---

vessel, blood vessel

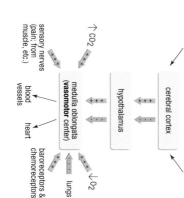

sensory nerves
(pain; from
muscle, etc.)

↑ CO_2

cerebral cortex

hypothalamus

medulla oblongata (**vasomotor** center)

blood
vessels

heart

baroreceptors &
chemoreceptors

↓ O_2

lungs

vasomotor
(vaso-motor)

1. Causing dilation or constriction of the blood vessels.
2. Denoting those nerves that have this action.

---

ventral, belly

ventrotomy
(ventro-tomy)

Transabdominal incision into the peritoneal cavity.

---

valve

valve

vagina

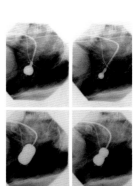

vaginosis
(vagin-osis)

Disease of the vagina.

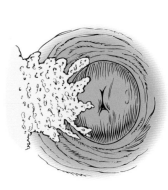

---

varix, varicose, varicosity

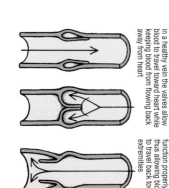

in a healthy vein the valves allow
blood to travel toward heart while
keeping blood from flowing back
away from heart

valves in varicose
veins no longer
function properly,
thus allowing blood
to travel back toward
extremities

varicosis
(varic-osis)

A dilated or varicose state of a vein or veins.

---

veins

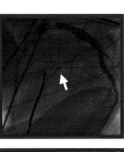
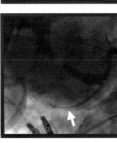

venography
(veno-graphy)

Radiographic demonstration of a vein, after the injection of contrast medium. Used to demonstrate blockage of a vein.

vertebr/o

Musculoskeletal System

Cardiovascular System

vestibul/o

Combining Form

The Senses

viscer/o

Gastrointestinal System

Combining Form

ventricul/o

Cardiovascular System

Combining Form

Prefix

Combining Form

Suffix

vesic/o, vesicul/o

Urinary System

Combining Form

Blood and the Immune System

Cardiovascular System

Endocrine System

Gastrointestinal System

General Terminology

Integumentary System

vir/o

General Terminology

Blood and the Immune System

Combining Form

Musculoskeletal System

Nervous System and Mental Health

Reproductive Systems

Respiratory System

The Senses

Urinary System

vertebra, vertebral

Word Building Example:

**vertebral column
(vertebr-al) column**

The series of vertebrae that extend from the cranium to the coccyx, providing support and forming a flexible bony case for the spinal cord.

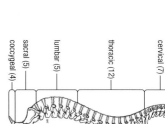

cervical (7)

thoracic (12)

lumbar (5)

sacral (5)

coccygeal (4)

ventricle

Word Building Example:

**ventriculostomy
(ventriculo-stomy)**

Establishment of an opening in a ventricle, usually through the floor of the third ventricle to the subarachnoid space to relieve hydrocephalus.

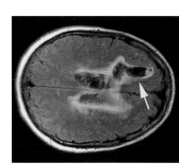

vestibule, vestibular apparatus (of ear)

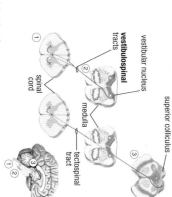

vestibulospinal tracts

vestibular nucleus

vestibulospinal

spinal cord

medulla

tectospinal tract

superior colliculus

vesica, vesicle

Word Building Example:

**vesiculate
(vesicul-ate)**

To become vesicular, characterized by or containing vesicles.

vestibulospinal
(vestibulo-spin-al)

A somatotopically organized fiber bundle originating from the lateral vestibular nucleus (nucleus of Deiters), which descends uncrossed into the anterior funiculus of the spinal cord lateral to the anterior median fissure.

the viscera

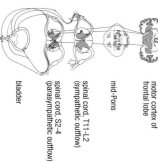

motor cortex of frontal lobe

mid-Pons

spinal cord, T11–L2 (sympathetic outflow)

spinal cord, S2–4 (parasympathetic outflow)

bladder

virus

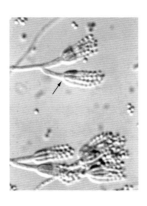

Word Building Example:

**virucidal
(viru-cidal)**

Destructive to a virus.

Word Building Example:

**visceromotor
(viscero-motor)**

Relating to or controlling movement in the viscera.

Card 794

viv/i

General Terminology

Card 793

vitr/o, vitre/o

The Senses

Combining Form

Prefix

Combining Form

Suffix

Card 796

xanth/o

General Terminology
Integumentary System

Combining Form

Card 795

vulv/o

Reproductive Systems
Urinary System

Combining Form

Blood and the Immune System

Cardiovascular System

Endocrine System

Gastrointestinal System

General Terminology

Integumentary System

Card 798

zo/o

Combining Form

Card 797

xiph/o

Musculoskeletal System

Combining Form

Musculoskeletal System

Nervous System and Mental Health

Reproductive Systems

Respiratory System

The Senses

Urinary System

living, alive

Word Building Example:

vivisection
(vivi-sect-ion)

Any cutting operation on a living animal for purposes of experimentation.

---

yellow, yellowish

Word Building Example:

xanthoma
(xanth-oma)

A yellow nodule or plaque, especially of the skin, composed of lipid-laden histiocytes.

---

animal life

Word Building Example:

zooglea
(zoo-glea)

In bacteriology, an old term for a mass of bacteria held together by a clear gelatinous substance.

---

vitreous

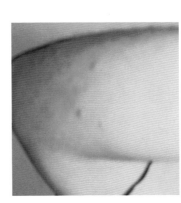

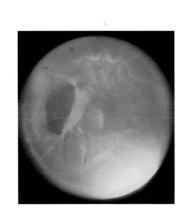

Word Building Example:

vitreoretinopathy
(vitreo-retino-pathy)

Retinopathy with vitreous complications.

---

vulva

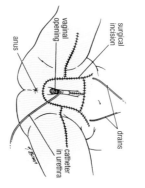

anus

vaginal opening

surgical incision

drains

catheter in urethra

Word Building Example:

vulvectomy
(vulv-ectomy)

Vulvar excision (partial, complete, or radical).

---

sword

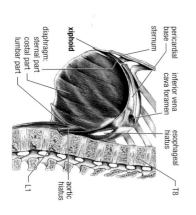

diaphragm:
sternal part
costal part
lumbar part

xiphoid

sternum

pericardial base

inferior vena cava foramen

esophageal hiatus

T8

aortic hiatus

L1

Word Building Example:

xiphoid process
(xiph-oid) process

The cartilage at the lower end of the sternum.